FUNDAMENTALS OF NURSING

Cally L. Davis

TAP

Toronto Academic Press

Fundamentals of Nursing

Cally L. Davis

Toronto Academic Press
224 Shoreacres Road
Burlington, ON L7L 2H2
Canada
www.tap-books.com
Email: orders@arclereducation.com

ISBN: 978-1-77469-794-8

ABOUT THE AUTHOR

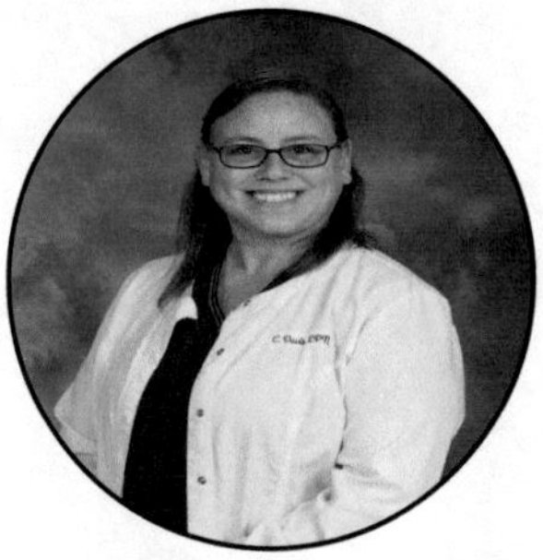

Cally is a Licensed Practical Nurse graduate from Wayne County Schools Career Center in Smithville, Ohio. She has 14 years of experience as an LPN for long term care facilities and outpatient surgical offices where she served as a charge nurse/office supervisor for up to six Certified Nursing Assistants and Medical Assistants. She is currently serving as an LPN at an elementary school enrolling approximately 500 students grades Pre-kindergarten to 5th grade.

Contents

3 Nursing Roles 45

4 Health and Wellness 71

5 Adult Nursing 97

List of Figures

List of Table

PREFACE

Nurses make up the backbone of the healthcare industry. Their roles as patient advocates and skilled care providers have never been more important in meeting the healthcare needs of an increasing number of patients. Nurses have long provided the general public with high-quality care. Professional respect in the medical community, on the other hand, was earned through years of lobbying, arranging, and, most importantly, academic advancement of the profession. Nurses were viewed as less integral members of a clinical care team 70 years ago (despite their many responsibilities), but they have fought for more recognition and now command much more respect and autonomy, enjoying an increasingly collaborative relationship with physicians and other healthcare professionals. Nurses today have more responsibility and independence. They have become an essential part of the healthcare team, which includes doctors, social workers, therapists, and others, to provide well-rounded, comprehensive patient care. Nurses have become linchpins in the essential communication between patients and providers because patients spend more time with them than with doctors or other healthcare professionals. The time nurses spend with patients gives them unique insights into their patients' wants and needs, behavior patterns, health habits, and concerns, making them valuable advocates in their care.

There is a vast amount of scientific literature on the issue. There have been a number of significant essays and books published on the subject that aim to critically analyze several individual contributions. This book focuses on an introduction to nursing education, its processes, principles of teaching and learning, the current roles of nurses in health care as well as the historical, ethical, political, social and legal aspects of nursing. There are eight chapters in the book. Thus, it can be used as a guide by student nurses and working nurses to recognize the nursing profession and to keep up with current developments. In this book, you will find all aspects of the nursing profession.

Chapter 1 introduces the nursing with history and development of nursing. It also explains nursing as a developing profession.

Chapter 2 focusses on the Nursing Process. The nursing process includes not just the behaviors required to complete tasks, but also critical thinking.

Chapter 3 sheds light on the roles of a nurse in the modern environment. It lists some implications of the new nursing roles. Additionally, presents a theory to understand new roles in nursing and highlights the influence of the biomedical model on nursing roles.

Chapter 4 presents an emphasis on Health and Wellness. To provide holistic care, the nurse must understand and respect each individual's concept of health and responses to sickness, as well as be knowledgeable about models of health and illness.

Chapter 5 is Adult Nursing that explores how to become an adult nurse. It also explains the role of nursing in adults in social care.

Chapter 6 is Gerontological Nursing. It starts with the history of gerontological nursing and the attitude towards aging and older adults. It also deals with principles of gerontological nursing, levels of geriatric care, and the role of a nurse.

Chapter 7 is Perioperative Nursing that deals with the surgical experience. It explains the nursing process for preoperative care, and teaches about surgical events and sensations.

Chapter 8 focuses on Legal and Ethical Aspects of Nursing. It deals with the ICN code of ethics and measures to prevent the above malpractice situations. In a democratic society, the legal system provides the foundation for interaction between all segments of the community.

–Author

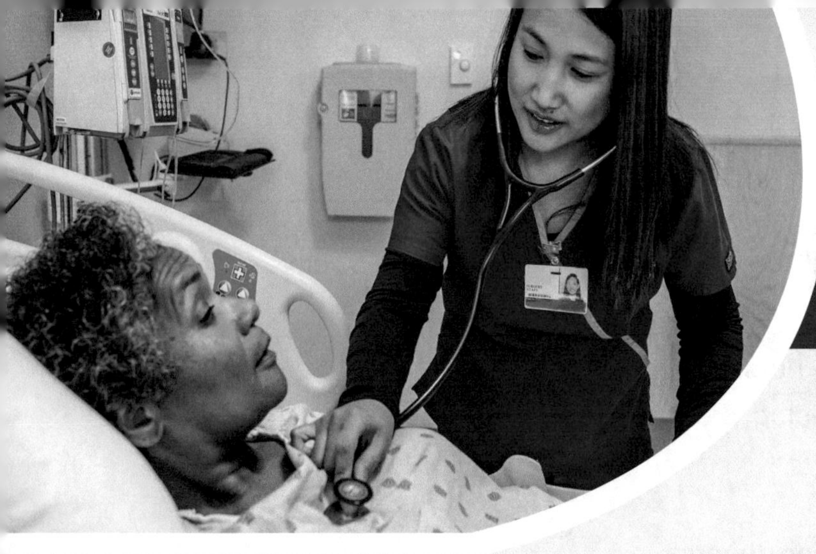

CHAPTER 1

INTRODUCTION TO NURSING

"Nurses are a unique kind. They have this insatiable need to care for others, which is both their greatest strength and fatal flaw."

—Jean Watson

INTRODUCTION

Nursing is a profession focused on helping people, families, and communities to attain, recover, and maintain optimum health and function from birth to old age. There are a variety of tasks involved in nursing care, ranging from complex technical processes to something as basic as holding a hand. Nursing combines both science and art. The science of nursing is the information base for the care provided, whereas the art of nursing is the skilled application of this knowledge to assist others in achieving their highest level of health and quality of life. This chapter explores an introduction to nursing.

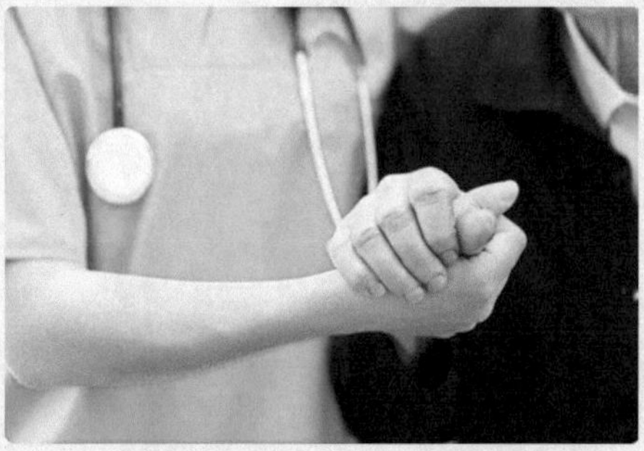

Learning Objectives

After completing the chapter, you will be able to accomplish the following:

- Definition of nursing
- History and development of nursing
- Explain nursing as a developing profession
- Philosophy of nursing theory
- Overview of nursing theory
- Elaborate the types of nursing theories

Key-terms

- Nursing
- Quality of life
- Optimal conditions
- Humanistic science
- Midwives
- Monasteries
- Formal socialization
- Informal socialization
- Organization socialization
- Self-awareness
- Nursing theory

DEFINITION OF NURSING

Different people have defined nursing differently. However, in this unit we will see some of the common definitions of nursing:

- Nursing is the provision of optimal conditions to enhance the person's reparative processes and prevent the reparative process from being interrupted.
- The practice of nursing is defined as diagnosing and treating human response to actual or potential health problems through such services as case finding, health teaching, health counseling; and provision of support to or restoration of life and well-being and executing medical regimes prescribed by licensed or otherwise legally authorized physicians or dentists.
- Nursing is directed toward meeting both the health and illness need and man who is viewed holistically as having physical, emotional, psychological intellectual, social and spiritual.
- Nursing is a humanistic science dedicated to compassionate concern with maintaining and promoting health, preventing illness and caring for and rehabilitating the sick and disabled.
- As a practice discipline nursing's scientific body of knowledge is used to provide an essential service to people, that is to promote the ability to affect health positively.

TIPS

Nursing is a deliberate action, a function of the practical intelligence of nurses and action to bring about humanely desirable conditions in persons and their environments.

HISTORY AND DEVELOPMENT OF NURSING

It is difficult to trace the exact origin of the nursing profession. However, moral action is the historical basis for the creation, evolution and practice of nursing.

Nursing in Ancient Civilization

The earliest records of ancient civilization contain few references to individuals who cared for the sick. During this time, views regarding the cause of disease were rooted in superstition and magic; hence, magical cures were frequently employed in treatment.

- To combat communicable diseases, the ancient Egyptians created community planning and strict hygienic regulations. The first recorded Nurses were seen here.

- The Babylonian culture contained references to jobs and procedures often performed by nurses. The Old Testament periodically mentions nurses as women who care for infants, the ill, and the dying, as well as midwives who assisted during pregnancy and childbirth.
- In mythology and reality, care for the ill and injured was advanced in ancient Rome. Despite the development of medicine as a science, there was no sign of a nursing basis being established.
- Ancient Greeks thought that their gods had remarkable healing abilities. Hippocrates was born around 460 BC and is considered the Father of Medicine. He demonstrated that disease had natural causes and not supernatural or supernatural causes. Physical evaluation, medical ethics, patient-centered treatment, and observation and reporting were initially recommended by Hippocrates. He stressed the significance of patient care, which contributed significantly to the foundation of nursing.
- In ancient India, male nurses staffed the earliest hospitals, while women acted as midwives and cared for ailing family members.

KEYWORD

Monasticism is a religious way of life in which one renounces worldly pursuits to devote oneself fully to spiritual work.

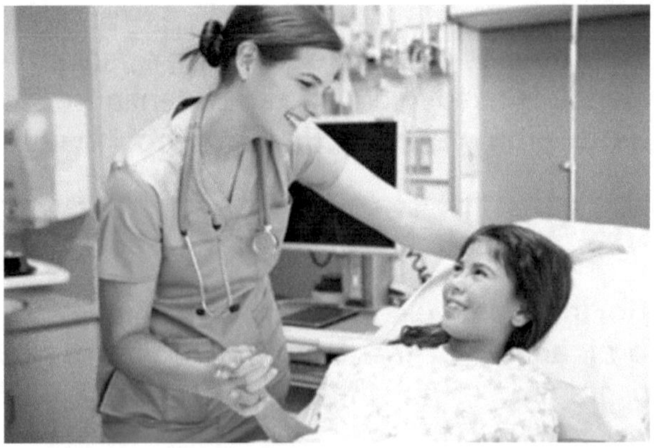

Nursing in the Middle Ages

Monasticism and other religious organizations provided the sole options for men and women to pursue careers in nursing during this period. The Christian precept "love your neighbor as thyself" has a great influence on the evolution of western nursing. Christ's tale of the Good Samaritan tending to an exhausted and hurt stranger developed the principle of compassion.

During the third and fourth centuries, numerous affluent Roman matrons, notably Marcella, Fabiola, and Paula, converted to Christianity and used their fortune to establish houses of care and healing for the destitute, the sick, and the homeless.

In the third century in Rome, women were not the sole givers of nursing care. There existed a group of men known as the Parabolani. This group of men provided care for the plague's sick and dying in Alexandria.

Dark Age of Nursing

During this time period, monasteries were shut down and women's participation in religious orders was practically eliminated. During this period, the few women who cared for the sick were prisoners or prostitutes with little or no nursing training. As a result, nursing was regarded as the most menial of all occupations and had little status and acceptance.

KEYWORD

Religious order is a lineage of communities and organizations of people who live in some way set apart from society in accordance with their specific religious devotion, usually characterized by the principles of its founder's religious practice.

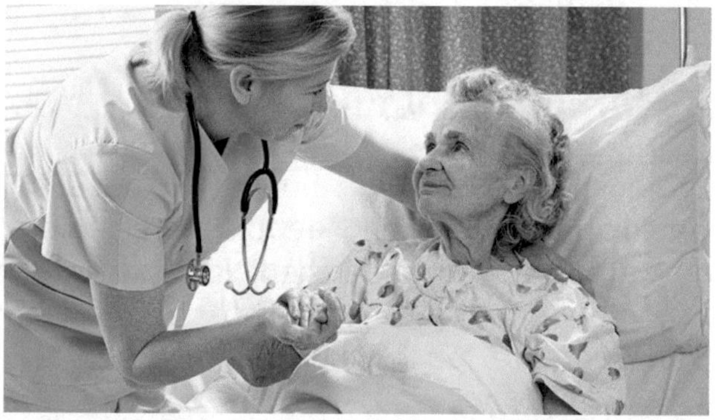

The Development of Modern Nursing

Three images have an impact on the evolution of modern nursing. The Ursuline Sisters of Quebec organized the initial nurse training. Theodore Flender revitalized the deaconess movement and founded a nursing school in Kaiserswerth, Germany. Elizabeth Fry founded the Nursing Sisters Institute. In the second half of the eighteenth century, however, Florence Nightingale, the founder of modern nursing, transformed the shape and direction of nursing and established it as a respectable profession. In 1820, she was born into an affluent and scholarly family. Despite objections from her family and a restrictive social code for an aristocratic young English woman to become a nurse, Florence Nightingale believed she was "called" by God to assist others and enhance the welfare of humanity. She got three months of training at Kaiserswerth in 1847. In 1853, she studied in Paris with a sister of charity, following which she returned to England to become the hospital's superintendent.

KEYWORD

Health Care Delivery Systems are the organizations that provide services to medical professionals like nurses, doctors, pharmacists, etc.

Nightingale strove to liberate nursing from the church's shackles. She viewed nursing as distinct from the church, yet she began her work as a result of her mystical experience.

Florence Nightingale was tasked with recruiting a troop of female nurses during the Crimean War. Mary Grant, a nurse from Jamaica, was the first nurse recruited to care for the Crimean war's wounded and sick. The accomplishments of Florence Nightingale throughout the war were so exceptional that the queen of England gave her the Order of Merit.

When she returned to England in 1860, she created the Florence Nightingale School of Nursing. It served as a model for other training institutions. Its alumni go abroad to lead hospitals and nurse training programs.

History of Nursing Ethiopia

In ancient Ethiopia, disease was thought to be a consequence of sins or magic. Most tribes and people had healers known as "Hakims" or "wegasha" who used medicinal plants and herbs to perform ceremonies and treat illness. Those in the Debre Libanos Monastery provided care for the sick and injured.

In Ethiopia, the health care delivery system was staffed by foreign nurses in the late 19th century, prior to the inception of nursing training. In 1917, Sister Karin Holmer traveled to Ethiopia as a qualified nurse.

In 1908, Emperor Menelik II founded the first government-sponsored public health services, which are now known as the ministry of public health, which was established in 1948. Ethiopia's first hospital, Menelik II, was constructed in 1909. Subsequently, his Imperial Majesty Haile Selassie I erected hospitals in many places, including Addis Ababa.

The first clinic was founded at the Eilet hot spring in Massawa, where sick individuals would bathe. 1948 saw the establishment of the Dejazmach Balcha Hospital through an arrangement with the Soviet Red Cross. The government of Ethiopia provided the structure. The Princess Tsehai Memorial Hospital was opened in 1951 as a homage to the British people as a symbol of their friendship with Ethiopia and with significant Ethiopian participation as a memorial to the late Princess Tsehai. It is now known as the Army Hospital.

Training of Medical Personnel

Before the Italian occupation, with exception of a mission school for midwives in Eritrea (the former province of Ethiopia), the only training in the public health personnel consisted of auxiliary medical training in several hospitals and missions.

The expansion of hospitals necessitated the training of Ethiopians to assist with hospital and clinic staffing. The Menelik II Hospital provided training facilities for medical auxiliary personnel as a first step.

Government and mission hospitals had been teaching dressers and other nursing orderlies for several years.

KEYWORD

Health Care Delivery Systems are the organizations that provide services to medical professionals like nurses, doctors, pharmacists, etc.

Ethiopian Nurses

Princess Tsehai, the emperor's youngest daughter was the first national nurse who graduated from Ormand Street Hospital, London. In 1948 the Ethiopian Red cross nursing school was established by his Imperial Majesty in the private Hospital Bet-Saida which later changed to Halie Selassie Hospital. Then during the Derg regime, this hospital changed its name to Yekatit 12 hospital, which still exists.

In 1950, the school of nursing was established at Empress Zewditu Memorial Hospital for male and female nurses. In March 1953, the first eight nurses graduated from the Ethiopian Red Cross of nursing and nine graduated from Empress Zewditu Memorial Hospital.

In 1951, two schools of Nursing were established: one at the Princess Tsehai memorial only for female nurses and the other one was in Nekemt at the TeferieMekonnen Hospital. In 1959 the post basic training started at princess Tsehai memorial hospital for midwifery nursing and four nurses graduated in 1960.

In 1954 the Gonder Health College and training center opened and gave training to community nurses. In 1958 fifteen (15) community nurses graduated from this center.

NURSING AS A DEVELOPING PROFESSION

Did you Know?

In the 19th and early 20th centuries, nursing was considered a women's profession, just as doctoring was a men's profession. With increasing expectations of workplace equality during the late 20th century, nursing became an officially gender-neutral profession, though in practice the percentage of male nurses remains well below that of female physicians in the early 21st century.

Profession and Professionalism

Nursing is a profession.

A profession is a calling that requires special knowledge and skilled preparation. A profession is generally distinguished from other kinds of occupation by:

a) Its requirement of prolonged specialized training acquiring a body of knowledge pertinent to the role to be performed and

b) An orientation of the individual to ward service, either to community or organization.

Criteria of a Profession

- Professional status is achieved when an occupation involves practice.
- A profession carries great individual responsibility and based on theoretical knowledge.
- The privilege to practice is granted only after the individual has completed a standardized program of highly specialized education and has demonstrated an ability to meet the standards for practice.
- The body of specialized knowledge is continually developed and evaluated through research.
- The members are self-organized and collectively assume the responsibility of establishing standards for education and practice.

Comparison between Profession and Occupation

Occupation	Profession
Training may occur on job	Education takes place in College and university
Length of training varies	Education is definite and prolonged

Value, beliefs and Ethics are not Prominent features of preparation	Value beliefs, and Ethics are integral part of preparation
Commitment & personal identification are strong	Commitment & personal Identification vary
Works are autonomous	Works are supervised
People unlikely to change jobs	Peoples often change Jobs
Accountability rests with individual	Accountability rests with employees

KEYWORD

Mission hospital means a private hospital sponsored by any religious body.

Professional Development

Professional development in nursing can be viewed in relation to specialized education, knowledge base, ethics, and autonomy.

Role of the Professional Nurse

- ***Care provider***: Caring /comforting. Involves knowledge and sensitivity to what matters and what is important to the client.
- ***Communicator / Helper***: Effective communication is an essential element of all helping professions, including nursing. It helps the client to explain the internal feeling.
- ***Teacher/educator***: This refers to activities by which the teacher helps the student to learn. The client will also need education based on the case.
- ***Counselor***: Counseling is a process of helping a client to recognize and cope with a stressful, psychological or a social problem, to develop improved interpersonal relationships and promote personal growth.
- ***Client advocate***: An advocate pleads the cause of others or argues or pleads for a cause or proposal.
- ***Change agent***: A change agent is a person or group who initiates changes or who assists others in making modifications in themselves or in the system.
- ***Leader***: Leadership is defined as a mutual process of inter personal influence through which the nurse helps a client make decision in establishing and achieving goals to improve the client's wellbeing.

- ***Manager***: Management defines a manager as who plans, gives direction, develops staff, monitoring operations, gives rewards fairly and represents both staff members and administration as needed.
- ***Researcher***: The majority of researchers in nursing are prepared at doctoral and post-doctoral levels. Although an increasing number of clinicians and nurses with a masters degree are beginning to practice it.

Remember

Enrolled nurses may initiate some oral medication orders with a specific competency now included in national curricula but variable in application by agency.

Nursing Education

- ***Practical Nurse Education***: Practical nursing has been in existence for many years. In the past, the practical nurse was the family, friends or community members who was called to the home during emergencies. These were lay people who gained such experience as they were self-taught. The first formal education in practical nursing was started in 1892. The duration of training was 3 months and students were called attendants. The curricula of practical nursing include child and elderly care, cooking and care of the sick at home.
- ***Licensed Practical Nursing***: This program is provided by high schools, community colleges, vocational schools, hospitals, and a variety of health agents. These programs usually last one year and provide both classroom and clinical experiences. In the end, the graduate takes the national council licensing examination to obtain a license as a practical or vocational nurse. In Ethiopia, the international licensed examination was given up until 1977. Later on, the national one was given and stopped in 1997.
- ***Registered Nursing***: In the United States, most basic education for registered nurses is provided in three types of programs, Diploma, Associate degree, and baccalaureate programs in Canada, the 2-years, 3- years or more diploma and baccalaureate programs prepare registered nurses.
- ***Diploma***: Today's diploma nursing programs have changed markedly from the original nightingale model, becoming hospital-based education programs that provide a rich clinical experience for nursing students these programs may last two or more years and are often associated with colleges or universities.
- ***Associate degree***: In 1980 as a solution to the acute

shortage of nurses that came about because of World War II. Associated degree programs are offered in the United States in junior colleges as well as in colleges and universities.

- ***Baccalaureate degree***: Although baccalaureate nursing education programs were established in universities in both United States and Canada in the early 1900s.In the 1960s the number of students enrolled in these programs increased markedly. In Ethiopia, this Program was started at Jimma University in 1993, later on, the Program continued in Della, Alemaya and Gonedr.
- ***Masters programs***: Master's programs generally take from 11/2 to 2 years to complete. In 1995 the numbers of nurses obtaining master's degrees increased. The mastered Programme has been proposed in September 2005 in Ethiopia.
- ***Doctoral programs***: Doctoral programs in nursing, which award the degree of doctor of nursing science (DNS). The program began in the 1960s in the United States.
- ***Continuing education***: - To formalize experiences designed to enlarge the knowledge or skills of practitioners.
- ***In service education***; - Program is administered by an employer; it is designed to update the knowledge or skills of employees.

Did you get it?

The World Bank's 2019 World Development Report on the future of work argues that professional development opportunities for those both in and out of work, such as flexible learning opportunities at universities and adult learning programs, enable labor markets to adjust to the future of work.

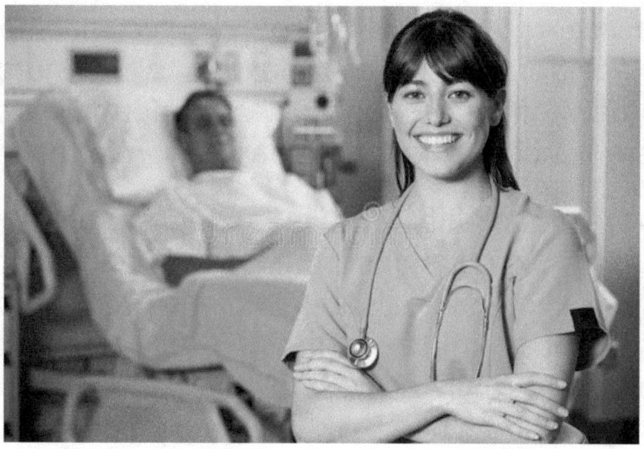

Socialization in Nursing

The nursing student internalizes the knowledge, skills, attitudes, beliefs, norms, culture, values, and ethical standards of nursing, incorporating them into their self-concept and conduct. Professional socialization is the process of internalization and formation of a professional identity. Socialization is the process by which an individual learns the norms of a group or society in order to participate effectively. Socialization is a process of mutual learning that takes place through interaction with others. It is considered that professional socialization in nursing occurs mostly, but not exclusively, during the student's time in basic nursing programs. It continues after graduation, when the student begins to practice nursing.

KEYWORD

Doctor of Nursing Science (D.N.S.) is an academic research degree awarded in a number of countries throughout the world as a terminal research degree in nursing.

ny new role is acquired through a combination of official and informal socializing. For example, little boys learn how to adopt the father role from what their own fathers teach them (formal socialization) and how they watch other fathers doing (informal socialization).

Formal socialization in Nursing contains topics the faculty wishes to teach, such as how to organize nursing care, do a physical examination on a healthy infant, and speak with a psychiatric patient.

Informal socialization includes lessons that occur inadvertently, such as overhearing a nurse instructs a young mother on how to care for her premature infant, participating in the student nurse association, or attending a nursing ethics committee meeting. Part of professional socialization is simply absorbing the culture of nursing, which consists of the rites, rituals, and valued behaviors of the profession.

This necessitates that students spend sufficient time with nurses in the workplace for adequate exposure to the nursing culture. The vast majority of nurses concur that informal socialization is frequently more effective and remembered than formal socialization.

Any new responsibility entails a degree of anxiety. When students' learning expectations conflict with educational realities, they frequently experience disappointment and frustration. What students believe they must learn and when they must learn it may differ from what really occurs? When patients observe nurses behaving in ways that deviate from their expectations of how nurses should behave, they are occasionally disillusioned. Students can more properly analyze the roots of their fear and more successfully control it if they are aware that these events may occur.

There is much more to socialization than the transmission of knowledge and skills. It serves to cultivate a shared nursing consciousness and is essential to maintaining the profession's vitality and dynamism. It is therefore not unexpected that a great lot of attention has been dedicated to this crucial process.

During socialization the nurse should:

- Value her/his own beliefs and practice while respecting the belief and practices of others.
- Respect the culture and religious beliefs of individuals.
- Become aware of the client's culture as described by the client and know the client's cultural values, beliefs, and behavior.
- Know what is right or wrong.

Therefore, the socialization process encompasses alterations in perception, knowledge, ability, attitudes, and values. As a nurse progresses and develops nursing knowledge, competence, attitudes, and values, he or she advances through five levels of proficiency. These levels of profiency are novice, advanced beginner, competent, proficient and expert.

- ***Stage 1 Novice:*** A novice may be a nursing student/ any nurse entering a clinical setting where that person has no experience and is governed by structured rules and protocols.
- ***Stage 2 Advanced beginner:*** Can demonstrate marginally accepted performance. The beginner has had experience with enough real situations to be aware of the meaningful aspect of the situation.
- ***Stage 3 Competent:*** The nurse who has been on the job in similar situations for 2 or 3 years manifests competence. Competence develops when the nurse consciously and deliberately plans nursing care and coordinates multiple complex care demands. Nursing competence provides a broad specification of nursing to cover the physical, psychological and spiritual care fields and serves as a bias for considering the objectives of training. The major components of competency include observation, interpretation, planning, action and evaluation.
- ***Stage 4 Proficient:*** The proficient nurse perceives a situation as a whole rather than just its individual aspects. The nurse focuses on long-term goals and is oriented toward managing the nursing care of a client rather than performing specific tasks.
- ***Stage 5 Expert:*** The expert nurse not only relies on rules,

KEYWORD

Formal socialization takes place in a structured environment, a school for example. In this environment an organized learning of skills, norms and information takes place.

guidelines, or maxims but also uses her/his understanding of a situation for an appropriate action.

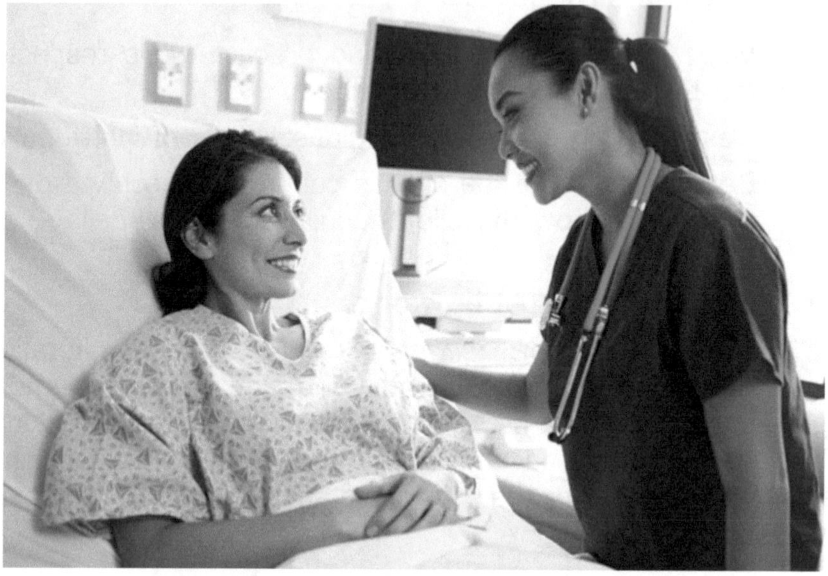

KEYWORD

Socialization is the process whereby an individual's standards, skills, motives, attitudes, and behaviors change to conform to those regarded as desirable and appropriate for his or her present and future role in any particular society.

Models of Professional Socialization

1. Cohen's stages of professional socialization

Stage I Unilateral dependence: Reliant on external authority, limited questioning or critical analysis. Students are unlikely to question or analyze critically the concepts teachers present because they lack the necessary background to do so.

Stage II Negatively/independence: cognitive rebellion, diminished reliance on external authority. Student's critical thinking abilities and knowledge bases expand

Stage III Dependence/mutuality: Reasoned appraisal, beings integration of facts and opinions following objective testing. Students evaluate the ideas of others. They develop an increasingly realistic appraisal process and learn to test concepts facts, ideas and models objectively.

Stage IV Interdependence collaborative decision-making: commitment to professional role; self-concept now includes professional role Identify. Students' needs for both independent and mutual (sharing jointly with others) aspects come together.

2. Hinshaw's stages of professional socialization

Hinshaw's stages of professional socialization is a potentially useful model describing the educational aspect of professional socialization.

Stage		Key behavior
I	Initial innocence	Initial image of nursing unaffected by reality
II	Incongruities	Initial expectations and reality collide, Questions carrier choice; may drop out
III	Identification	Observes behavior of experienced nurses
IV	Role simulation	Practices observed behavior; way feed unnatural in role
V	Vacillation	Old image and conflict with new professional image
VI	Internalization	Acceptance and comfort with new role

KEYWORD

Critical thinking is the analysis of available facts, evidence, observations, and arguments in order to form a judgment by the application of rational, skeptical, and unbiased analyses and evaluation.

Organization Socialization

Organization socialization is the process by which a person develops an appreciation for the values, talents, anticipated behaviors, and social knowledge necessary for assuming an organizational role and engaging as a member of the organization.

Through socialization, the organization aims to establish high levels of individual performance, which will have a favorable effect on group and organizational outputs.

Each organization is an evolving social structure with its own set of values, ideas, frictions, conflicts, and coalitions of allies. The purpose of orientation is to help the new employee to enter the system wisely and successfully adapt.Socialization entails an introduction to group norms, i.e., the respected ideals and patterns of behavior.

Group norms are developed as a nurse's attempt to defuse a potentially explosive conflict of interest; the two competing objectives are:

1. A desire for companionship and peer acceptance, and
2. A human yearning for autonomy and individuality. Positive (supportive), negative (obstructive), or neutral group norms are possible (ineffectual)

The student nurses require organization orientation. The job of the organization is to merge individual and organizational demands so as to sustain the individual's integrity and self-confidence as well as the organization's effectiveness and cohesion.

International and National Nursing Association

- Associations are organizations of persons with common interests.
- As the number of nurses increased the activities and problems in connection with work also increased.
- A professional association is an association of practitioners who judge one another as professionally competent and who banded together to perform social functions that they cannot perform in their separate capacities as an individual.

Nursing Association

TIPS

As each person is unique, so too is each organization. The specific objective of orientation is the combination of these match-less entities without sacrificing one and enhancing both.

The nursing association must perform the following five functions for the preservation and development of its profession

- Defining and regulating the profession through setting and enforcing standards of education and of education and practice for generalists and specialists.
- Developing the knowledge base for practice in its broadest and narrowest components.
- Transmitting values norms, knowledge, and skill to nursing students, new graduates and members of the profession for application in practice.
- Communicating and advocating the value and contribution of the field to several publics and constituencies.
- Attending to the social and general welfare of their member. Professional associations give their member social and moral support to perform their roles as professionals and cope with professional problems.

International Council of Nurses (ICN)

- The International Council of Nurses (ICN) was established in 1899.
- Nurses from Great Britain, the United States, and Canada were among the founding members.

- The Council is a federation of national nurses associations, such as the American Nursing Association (ANA) and Canadian Association for Nurses (CAN).
- In 1993, 111 national nurses associations representing 1.4 million nurses worldwide were affiliated with the ICN.
- The ICN provides an organization through which members of the National Nursing Association can work together to promote the health of people and the care of the sick.

The Objectives of ICN are:

- To improve the standers and states of Nursing
- To promote the development of a strong National Nurses' Association
- To serve as the authoritative voice for nurses and the nursing profession worldwide.

Remember

Tactics used in this process include formal meetings, lectures, videos, printed materials, or computer-based orientations that outline the operations and culture of the organization that the employee is entering into. This process is known in other parts of the world as an 'induction' or training.

PHILOSOPHY OF NURSING THEORY

Personal values that guide and shape our attitudes, behaviors, and decisions in all aspects of life generate principled conduct. Making ethical decisions involves self-awareness and an understanding of ethical theories and principles. Such self-awareness includes the knowledge of our values and priorities. Personal values and moral growth influence views and decisions. This section analyzes the relationship between nursing beliefs, values, and philosophies. Therefore, readers are urged to examine their own values, perspectives, and tendencies, as well as those of others and the circumstances in which they find themselves, in relation to various decision-making processes.

Beliefs, Values and Philosophy of Nursing

Beliefs

A belief is the intellectual acknowledgment that something is true or correct. Beliefs are also known as convictions and creeds. Beliefs are opinions that may be accurate or untrue in reality. They are founded on acquired and substantiated attitudes. Generally, beliefs are handed from one generation to the next.

Because the practice of nursing frequently challenges nurses' views, it is crucial to recognize and comprehend one's beliefs in nursing. Although this may cause temporary agony, it is ultimately beneficial since it compels nurses to thoroughly examine their views. They have to answer the question: "Is this something I really believe, or have I accepted it because some influential person (such as a parent or teacher) said it?" Abortion, living wills, the freedom to die, the right to refuse treatment, alternative lifestyles, and related concerns confront every member of modern society.

Remember

Professional nurses must develop and refine their beliefs about these and many other issues.

Beliefs manifest themselves through attitudes and actions. Observing nurses' interactions with patients, their families, and other nurses reveals something about their beliefs. Every day, nurses come into contact with individuals whose beliefs differ from, or are diametrically opposed to, their own. Effective nurses appreciate the necessity of adopting a nonjudgmental stance toward patients' religious views. A nurse with a nonjudgmental attitude makes every attempt to communicate neither approval nor condemnation of patients' opinions and respects the right of each individual to hold those ideas.

Categories of Beliefs

People often use the terms beliefs and values interchangeably. Even experts disagree about whether they differ or are the same. Although they are related, beliefs and values are different.

There are three main categories of beliefs:

- ***Descriptive or existential beliefs***: are those that are shown to be true or false. An example of a descriptive belief is: "The sun will come up each morning."
- ***Evaluative beliefs***: are those in which there is a judgment about good or bad. The belief that "Dancing is immoral" is an example of an evaluative belief.
- ***Prescriptive (encouraged) and proscriptive (prohibited) beliefs***: are those in which certain actions are judged to be desirable or undesirable. The belief "Every citizen of voting age should vote in every election" is a prescriptive belief, whereas the belief "People should not engage in sexual intercourse outside of marriage" is a proscriptive belief. Prescriptive and proscriptive beliefs are closely related to values.

Values

Values are the societal beliefs, ideas, or standards maintained by a person, group, or class that give life meaning and purpose. A value is an abstract depiction of what is appropriate, valuable, or desired. Values are what individuals deem desirable and consist of the subjective attribution of value to conduct.

Despite the fact that many individuals are unaware of it, values help them make both little, day-to-day decisions and large, life-altering ones. In the same way that beliefs influence nursing practice, so do values, frequently without the nurses' conscious awareness. Everything we do, every decision we make, and every action we take is dependent on the beliefs, attitudes, and values we have consciously and unconsciously selected. Nursing is a manifestation of the nurse's values through behavior.

People with uncertain values are lacking in direction, perseverance, and decision-making ability. Effective nurses must possess a robust set of professional nursing values since much of nursing requires a strong sense of direction, perseverance, and the capacity to make smart judgments quickly and regularly.

KEYWORD

Self-awareness is the ability to focus on yourself and how your actions, thoughts, or emotions do or don't align with your internal standards.

Types of Values

- *Personal Values*: Most people drive some values from the society in which they live. E.g.: self-worth, sense of humor, honesty, fairness and love
- *Professional values:* are reflections of personal values. They are acquired during socialization into nursing. Some of the important values of nursing are:
  - Strong commitment to service
  - Belief in the dignity and worth of each person
  - Commitment to education
  - Autonomy

Remember

Primary prevention relates to general knowledge applied in client assessment and intervention in identifying and reducing or mitigating possible or actual risk factors associated with environmental stressors to prevent a possible reaction.

Values Clarification

Nurses as well as people in other helping professions need to understand their values. This is the first step in self-awareness, which is important in maintaining a nonjudgmental approach to patients.

Importance of Value Clarification for Nurses in Professional Practice

Value clarification in nursing:

- Provides a basis for understanding how and why we react and respond in decision-making situations.

- Enables us to acknowledge similarities and differences in values when interacting with others which ultimately promotes more effective communication and care
- Enables nurses to be more effective in facilitating the nursing process with others

KEYWORD

Decision making is the process of making choices by identifying a decision, gathering information, and assessing alternative resolutions.

Impact of Institutional Values on Nurses

Nurses must be aware of both the stated and unstated values in their work environments. Because choosing employment entails a commitment to the institution's value system, nurses should discover congruence between their own and institutional ideals.

Values Govern Nursing's Social Policy statement

The behaviors of a group, such as the nursing profession, reveal its collective identity. These acts result from a set of values and decisions, and by analyzing the actions of groups, their fundamental values can be deduced.

The values of the profession are articulated by organized nurses. This is accomplished by the periodic publication of a document intended to explain nursing's link with society and its responsibilities to persons who receive nursing care.

TIPS

Environmental interaction refers to the ways in which living organisms, including humans, interact with and are influenced by their surrounding environment. This interaction can take various forms and occur at different levels, ranging from individual organisms to ecosystems.

Philosophies of Nursing

Nursing philosophies are declarations of views about nursing and expressions of nursing values that serve as mental and behavioral foundations. Most nursing philosophies are founded on views about people, the environment, health, and nursing.

Every nurse has a philosophy consisting of a set of beliefs upon which nursing actions are based.

Personal and professional ideologies of nurses interact intimately and impact professional conduct. An important aspect of nursing philosophy is that they are dynamic and evolve throughout time. Developing a nursing philosophy is not only an academic requirement for accreditation. Having a documented philosophy can aid nurses in the everyday discussions they are required to have regarding nursing practice.

OVERVIEW OF NURSING THEORY

NThe nursing theory attempts to describe or explain the phenomenon of nursing. Nursing theory differentiates nursing from other disciplines and activities.

Theories are general concepts used to explain, predict, control, and understand commonly occurring events. Theories provide a method of classifying and organizing data in a logical, meaningful manner. A theory is a set of systematically interrelated concepts or hypotheses that seeks to explain and predict phenomena.

KEYWORD

Collective identity refers to the shared definition of a group that derives from its members' common interests, experiences, and solidarities.

There have been three reasons for the interest in theory:

- Theory development contributes to knowledge building and is seen as a means of establishing nursing as a profession.
- The growth and enrichment of theory in and of itself is an important goal of nursing, as a scholarly discipline, to pursue.
- Theory helps practicing nurses categorize and understand what is going on in nursing practice. It helps them to predict a client's response to nursing services and is helpful in clinical decision-making.

TYPES OF NURSING THEORIES

General Systems Theory

A system is a collection of interacting elements with the shared goal of contributing to the system's overall objective. Always, the whole is larger than the sum of its parts.

Systems are hierarchical in structure and are built of interdependent subsystems that work together in such a way that a change to one part may influence other subsystems as well as the entire system. Boundaries isolate systems from both one another and their surroundings.

A system interacts with and responds to its environment by processes that enter the system (input) or are transferred to the environment (output). An open system permits the unrestricted flow of energy, matter, and information across system boundaries. Open systems maintain equilibrium via feedback. Understanding systems theory allows nurses to evaluate the interplay between the input, output, and throughput processes. The system approach enables nurses to view the individual client, his or her family, and the community as a whole.

Neuman Systems Theory

KEYWORD

Nursing services means those services pertaining to the preventive, curative, and restorative aspects of nursing care that are performed by or under the supervision of a registered professional nurse.

The Neuman systems theory is an open systems concept consisting of two essential components: stress and response to it. Both harmful and helpful stimuli act on the system, which strives to maintain equilibrium or homeostasis.

Nursing is an integral aspect of the health care system and the social structure that surrounds it. The reciprocal interaction between nursing and system components contributes to the proper functioning and evolutionary survival of the entire system. The nurse evaluates entropy and negentropy to guide her/his interventions, which try to combat entropy through evolutionary adaptation, restoring and maintaining equilibrium between forces or stressors. The nurse evaluates the aspects that influence a person's perceptual field, including the significance a stressor has for the client and the factors in his/her own perceptual field that influence evaluation and caregiving.

Roy Adaptation Theory

This theory defines nursing as the practice of promoting the adaptation of a person's four subsystems (physiologic, self-concept, role function, interdependence). Within the nursing process, the nurse strives to change or maintain stimuli affecting adaption. Nursing assessment focuses on two units of analysis: the person's system and interaction with the environment, whereas intervention focuses on the alteration of system or environment components.

Orem's Self-Care Nursing Theory

The model is centered on the idea of self-care. Orem defines nursing as the creative endeavor of one individual to assist another. Nursing is a helping system that can be wholly compensatory; that is, the client is unable to achieve self-care and therefore has health deviation self-care requirements; partially compensatory where both nurse and client work to achieve self-care; or supportive, educative, where the client is able to perform, or can and should perform self-care but does not do so independently.

Rogers Model of the Science of Unitary Man

Martha Rogers developed a model based on systems theory. She developed her model around four components, which she called:

- Universe of open systems
- Energy fields
- Pattern and organization and
- Four dimensionality

Using this model one can focus on client environment interaction and see the client as functioning interdependently with others and the environment. The nurse's goal is to promote holistic health and environment interaction in order to maximize client health potential.

KEYWORD

Open system is one in which there is an exchange of both matter and energy with its surroundings.

Johnson Behavioral Systems Model

Johnson argues that nursing care should focus on caring for the whole patient in order to enable the effective and efficient behaviors required to prevent sickness. Johnson considers nursing to be distinct from medicine. She views the job of nursing as complementary to the role of medicine.

This model emphasizes that in order to sustain homeostasis, both the internal and external environments of the system must be ordered and predictable. If the subsystems are out of balance, there will be tension and disequilibrium. As a component of the external environment, nursing can assist the patient in regaining equilibrium.

REVIEW QUESTIONS

1. What do you understand by nursing?
2. Discuss how a philosophy of nursing influences nursing practice
3. What is the importance of theory development in nursing?
4. Discuss some of the commonly used theories in nursing.
5. You are appointed to a position of a Matron in a new hospital, and are asked to formulate a philosophy- how do you do it?

MULTIPLE CHOICE QUESTIONS

1. Which phrase best describes the science of nursing?
   a. The skilled application of knowledge
   b. The knowledge base for care
   c. Hands-on care, such as giving a bath
   d. Respect for each individual patient

2. Which nurse in history is credited with establishing nursing education?
   a. Clara Barton
   b. Lillian Wald
   c. Lavinia Dock
   d. Florence Nightingale

3. What historic event in the 20th century led to an increased emphasis on nursing and broadened the role of nurses?
   a. Religious reform
   b. Crimean War
   c. World War II
   d. Vietnam War

4. A school nurse is teaching a class of junior-high students about the effects of smoking. This educational program will meet which of the aims of nursing?
   a. Promoting health
   b. Preventing illness
   c. Restoring health
   d. Facilitating coping with disability or death

5. Which of the following nursing degrees prepares a nurse for advanced practice as a clinical specialist or nurse practitioner?
   a. LPN

b. ADN
c. BSN
d. Master's

Answers to Multiple Choice Questions

1. (b) 2. (d) 3. (c) 4. (b) 5. (d)

REFERENCES

1. American Nurses Association (ANA). (2003). Nursing: Scope and standards of practice: Professional development. Washington, DC: Author.
2. American Nurses Association (ANA). (2005). Core issues. Washington, DC: Author.
3. American Nurses Association (ANA). (2009). Considering nursing? Available http://www.nursingworld.org/EspeciallyForYou/ StudentNurses.aspx
4. Blais, K., Hayes, J., &Kozier, B. (2005). Professional nursing practice: Concepts and perspectives (5th ed.). Upper Saddle River, NJ: Pearson Prentice Hall.
5. Buerhaus, P. (2007). Dealing with reality: Confronting the global nursing shortage. Reflections on Nursing Leadership, Fourth Quarter, 6 p.
6. D'Antonio, P. (2004). Women, nursing, and baccalaureate education in 20th century America. Journal of Nursing Scholarship, 36(4), 379–384.
7. D'Antonio, P. (2006). History for a practice profession. Nursing Inquiry, 13(4), 242–248.
8. Dolan, J. A., Fitzpatrick, M. L., & Herrmann, E. K. (1983). Nursing in society: A historical perspective. Philadelphia: W. B. Saunders.
9. Donley, R., Sr. (2005). Challenges for nursing in the 21st century. Nursing Economics, 23(6), 312–318.
10. Ellis, J., & Hartley, C. (2007). Nursing in today's world: Challenges, issues, trends (9th ed.). Philadelphia: Lippincott Williams & Wilkins.
11. Fairman, J. (2008). Context and contingency in the history of post-World War II nursing scholarship in the United States. Journal of Nursing Scholarship, 40(1), 4–11.
12. International Council of Nurses. (2002). The ICN definition of nursing. Geneva: ImprimeriesPopulaires.
13. Kalisch, P. A., &Kalisch, B. J. (2004). American nursing: A history. Philadelphia: Lippincott Williams & Wilkins.
14. Lauridsen, B. (2005). Stepping stones on which today's nursing was built. Nursing BC, 37(2), 5.
15. National Council of State Boards of Nursing. (2008). Nurse licensure compact administration, Participating states in the NLC. Available at https://www.ncsbn.org/158.htm

16. Nightingale, F. (1992). Notes on nursing: What it is and what it is not. (Commemorative ed.). Philadelphia: J. B. Lippincott.
17. Pender, N. J., Murdaugh, C., & Parsons, M. A. (2006). Health promotion in nursing practice (5th ed.). Upper Saddle River, NJ: Prentice Hall.
18. Price-Spratlen, L., & Mahoney, M. (2006). February, Black History Month: A time to review nursing's past, present, and future. Washington Nurse, 36(1), 12–13.
19. Smeltzer, C. H., Vlasses, F. R., & Robinson, C. R. (2005). A look back . . . "If we only had a nurse" . . . historical view of a nurse shortage. Journal of Nursing Care Quality, 20(2), 190–192.
20. Stanley, D. (2007). Lights in the shadows: Florence Nightingale and others who made their mark. Contemporary Nurse, 24(1), 45–51.
21. U.S. Department of Health and Human Services, Office of Disease Prevention and Health Promotion. (2000). Healthy people 2010.
22. Wall, B. M. (2008). Celebrating nursing history. American Journal of Nursing, 108(6), 26–29.
23. West, R. A., Griffith, G. P., &Iphofen, R. (2007). A historical perspective on the nursing shortage. MEDSURG Nursing, 16(2), 124–130.

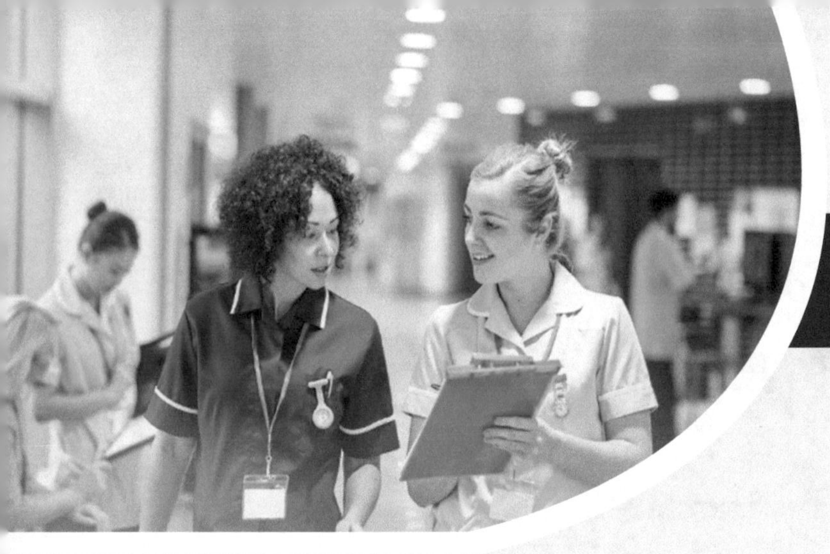

CHAPTER 2

INTRODUCTION TO THE NURSING PROCESS

"Constant attention by a good nurse may be just as important as a major operation by a surgeon."

—Dag Hammarskjöld

INTRODUCTION

The primary objective of nursing is to assist individuals in meeting their basic and advanced requirements. Specific interactions, including communication, observation, support, education, and the provision of care, result from meetings with clients. Nurses promote and encourage individuals to maintain healthy lifestyles and assist them in resolving health issues. They provide care to clients through the nursing process by combining scientific problem-solving techniques with critical thinking skills.

The Nursing Process is a fundamentally distinct problem-solving method that emphasizes the contrasts between licensed personnel (RN and LPN/LVN) and non-licensed personnel (CNA, NA, UAP). The nursing process includes not just the behaviors required to complete tasks, but also critical thinking. In other words, unlicensed workers must be able to measure vital signs. In addition to knowing how to take vital signs, a certified nurse must also understand their significance and the relationship between the numbers obtained and the patient's condition.

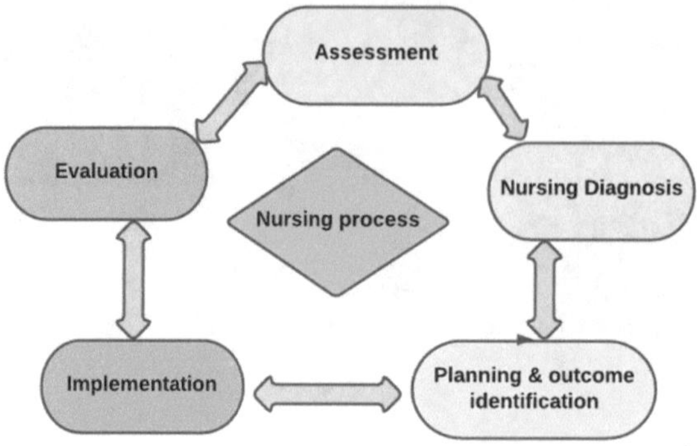

Learning Objectives

After completing the chapter, you will be able to accomplish the following:

- Discuss about problem-solving
- Define critical thinking
- Explain the nursing process

Key-terms

- Problem-solving
- Healthcare researchers
- Critical thinking
- Nursing care plan
- Auscultation
- Intravenous (IV) fluid therapy

PROBLEM-SOLVING

Problem-solving is the fundamental ability to recognize a problem and take action to resolve it. Common sense is useful in solving a variety of issues. However, when a problem is complex or difficult to define, you may need to employ other, more formal problem-solving techniques.

Trial and Error

Trial-and-error problem-solving is an experimental way of determining which solutions are effective and which are not. Because the experimenter lacks sufficient knowledge to predict results, the results are generally unknown until the experiment is conducted. On occasion, you employ trial and error to address ordinary problems. Consider your predicament if you are allergic to an unidentified ingredient in hand lotion, but also suffer from dry skin and want to moisturize your hands. You try a certain brand, but develop a rash. You try a different brand with identical results.

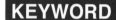

KEYWORD

Allergic reactions are inappropriate responses of the immune system to a normally harmless substance.

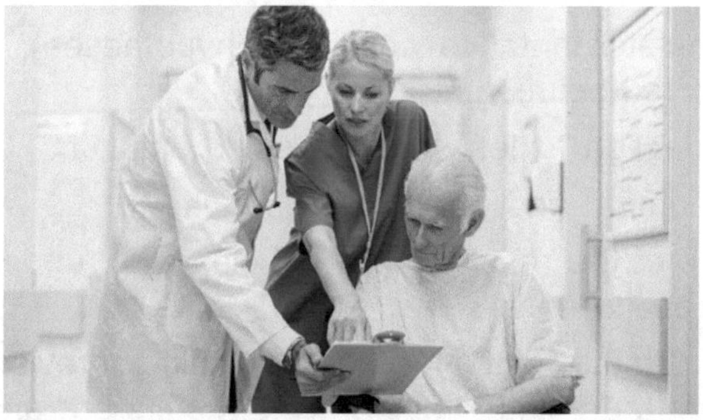

These trials result in errors: The lotions continue to cause an allergic response. Eventually, you find a brand that works without causing a rash, and your trial is successful.

In laboratory investigations, a sort of trial-and-error experimentation is utilized when comparing multiple solutions to a problem. The elimination of toxic or ineffective solutions until the discovery of beneficial ones. In other cases, trial and error is utilized when unexpected findings that may be advantageous to another problem arise. For instance, minoxidil (Rogaine) was initially promoted as a hypertension medication. The unexpected result of hair growth, however, led to the testing and development of pharmacological formulations for the treatment of hair loss.

Remember

The nursing process can be used to identify not only the client's actual problems, but also potential problems.

Numerous advancements in contemporary healthcare have evolved from this form of testing; nevertheless, trial and error must be utilized with caution when working with people due to the potential for adverse outcomes. Researchers set stringent standards to preserve the safety and well-being of persons, and they conduct trial-and-error experiments only with the consent and knowledge of the subject.

Scientific Problem-Solving

Today's society prefers that ailing individuals receive only proven safe and effective treatments. Therefore, healthcare providers rely on already established evidence to judge the safety of a treatment. Scientists and healthcare researchers analyze problems and arrive at answers using a methodical procedure. This strategy, known as scientific problem-solving, enables researchers to identify the safest and most effective remedies for sickness or malfunction. The following are the seven steps of scientific problem-solving:

- Identify the problem.
- Gather information relative to the problem.
- Formulate tentative solutions (hypotheses); choose the preferred solution.
- Plan action to test the suggested solution.
- Experiment and observe the results.
- Interpret the results (draw conclusions); understand what the results mean.
- Evaluate the solution, either concluding or revising the study to test the solution again if the results are unsatisfactory.

CRITICAL THINKING

Unless you have a scientific background, you usually solve problems without using trial-and-error or scientific problem-solving. Critical thinking is a complex combination of inquiry, knowledge, intuition, logic, experience, and common sense. This way of thinking enables you to comprehend the significance of various hints and find speedy solutions to challenging issues. Critical thinking is neither a trial-and-error process nor an organized scientific method for solving problems. Certain elements of critical thinking are vital for solving healthcare challenges. When you think critically, you examine facts and compare these facts with information you already know, thereby being actively curious and critiquing ideas for reasonableness.

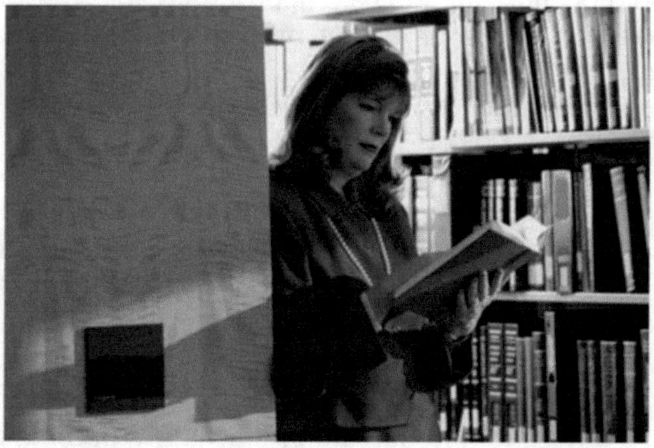

Figure 2.1: Critical thinking utilizes previous knowledge, research, and analysis, as well as common sense, to solve problems.

You form concepts or ideas that are mental representations of reality. You are logical and rational, constantly seeking to comprehend the full scenario. You may think without technique or structure, but you do not leap to conclusions. As a critical thinker, you establish your own opinions and ideas rather than accepting those of others without question. You become an adaptable individual with an open mind. You also utilize your ideas and ingenuity to acquire information and draw conclusions in a methodical manner (Figure 2.1).

Consider a basic illustration of how you employ critical thinking when faced with a challenge. One morning you discover that your automobile keys are not in their normal spot. You have barely 30 minutes to reach class for a mandatory exam. What do you do initially? You probably search furiously once again, but pause to consider where else you could have lost your keys. Perhaps you retrace your steps from the day before, when you had your keys last. You question, "Where was I? What were my actions? Have I forgotten them in a pocket? What was my attire? By asking yourself logical questions, memorizing the facts, forming a mental image of your actions, and possibly following an intuition about the location of the keys, you may be able to swiftly solve your dilemma and locate your keys. If you cannot discover them within an acceptable amount of time, you begin to consider alternative solutions to the problem of attending the needed examination. This is referred to as critical thinking: memorizing facts, employing logic, asking crucial questions, constructing an image in one's mind, and assessing all information.

Most client care difficulties have several plausible causes and many probable answers. When you think critically, it is easier to comprehend the nature and scope of problems. You are able to make decisions that are logical, appropriate for a certain client, and effective in fixing a particular problem.

THE NURSING PROCESS

Although you will employ critical thinking throughout your nursing career, it does not provide a framework for systematically and consciously solving problems, a vital safeguard in healthcare. As a nurse, you combine critical thinking with a scientific approach to problem-solving to identify client problems and provide structured, meaningful, and efficient treatment. This mental and behavioral framework is known as the nursing process. The nursing process is a unique technique of considering how to provide care for patients. The nursing process is also described as a systematic method that directs the nurse and client as they together (1) determine the need for nursing care, (2) plan and implement the care, and (3) evaluate the results.

Did you Know?

The nursing process is a modified scientific method. Nursing practice was first described as a four-stage nursing process by Ida Jean Orlando in 1958.

You will utilize the nursing process framework throughout your nursing profession, but especially during your nursing education. The nursing process is the procedure for identifying and treating client care issues. To maintain uniformity across all nursing staff, set care guidelines for each client using the nursing process.

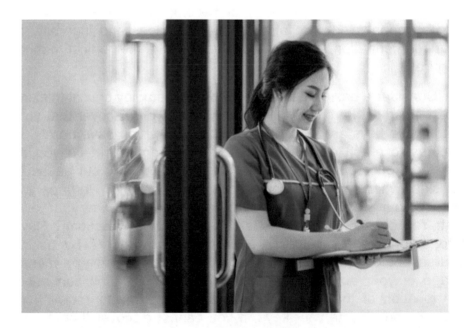

Traditionally, these recommendations are formulated in a framework known as a nursing care plan (NCP). Modern, clinical nursing units may substitute alternative terminology for the nursing care plan, such as critical pathways, idea mapping, or clinical pathways, but the process of thinking through the nursing process is essentially the same regardless of the language used. The nursing process framework permits the development of tailored plans of care for each client by identifying what is suitable and desirable for that individual. In practice, Nursing Care Plan 1 describes a patient with pneumonia who is an elderly woman. The care plan facilitates more efficient time management while providing care. Because the nursing care plan is available for other nurses to use as well, it provides consistency in care.

Remember

Remember that every time you create a care plan, you're enhancing your critical thinking and nursing expertise. Also, keep in mind that every time you execute your strategy, you are performing nursing duties. Eventually, this mental and physical process becomes automatic.

Effective application of the nursing process permits identification of both existing and potential problems. Potential issues are those that could be avoided or that the customer is at risk of developing. The ability to anticipate difficulties can prevent both unpleasant and expensive complications. The nursing procedure also allows you to judge if the client benefited from your nursing care.

Working through the nursing process framework frequently as you learn to identify and address client needs will help you develop critical thinking and problem-solving abilities. As you construct nursing care plans, you will frequently apply the steps of the nursing process.

The nursing process framework has been utilized in the United States and Canada for more than 50 years as a guide for assessing client needs and providing care, but its application varies by region. Its format may differ between types of healthcare facilities and be contingent on the availability of personnel. In certain areas of practice, registered nurses are more likely to diagnose patients, establish overall care objectives, and plan treatment. In other settings, licensed practical nurses also diagnose and implement treatment plans. Determine what your job (as a student and a graduate) is anticipated to be in your particular healthcare facility.

Steps in the Nursing Process

The nursing process has specific steps in which you work with the client to plan and to carry out effective nursing care:

- ***Nursing Assessment:*** the systematic and continuous collection of data (see Figure 2.2)

- ***Nursing Diagnosis:*** the statement (or label) of the client's actual or potential problem
- ***Planning:*** the development of goals for care and possible activities to meet them
- ***Implementation:*** the giving of actual nursing care
- ***Evaluation:*** the measurement of the effectiveness of nursing care

TIPS

The nursing process provides individualized care that is accountable.

Characteristics of the Nursing Process

The nursing process steps lead to certain outcomes. The efficacy of the nursing process is dependent on the features outlined in the following sections.

The five steps of the nursing process are remarkably similar to the steps of scientific problem-solving. Table 2.1 illustrates the relationship between nursing process steps and scientific problem-solving approach concepts.

Table 2.1: The Nursing Process Compared With Scientific Problem-Solving

STEPS IN SCIENTIFIC PROBLEM-SOLVING	RELATED STEPS IN THE NURSING PROCESS	ACTIVITIES TO PERFORM
Gather information relative to the problem. Identify the problem.	Nursing assessment Nursing diagnosis	Identify priorities; collect data; update database. Recognize and label significant data; recognize patterns or clusters; identify strengths and problems; reach conclusions; validate observations; write diagnostic statements.
Formulate tentative solutions; describe possible solutions; choose preferred solutions; plan ways to test suggested solution.	Planning	Identify priorities; establish expected outcomes or goals; anticipate nursing interventions; prepare to document specific actions that will reach outcomes/ goals by stating specific timeline for the plan (i.e., set short-term and long-term goals to suit the needs of the client)

Test solutions.	Implementation and interventions	Take actions that are necessary to achieve goals. Adjust actions as conditions change. Monitor and report results of assessment, goals, and interventions to other healthcare team members.
Evaluate the solution; evaluate the results.	Evaluation	Analyze (use critical thinking skills) the client's responses to the problem, goals, and actions. Identify factors that contributed to success or failure of the nursing care plan's outcomes or goals. Re-evaluate and reassess; continue with nursing process in a cyclic manner.
Formulate another tentative solution.	Revision and re-evaluation	Revise plan for future nursing care based on new assessments and data.

KEYWORD

Prioritization is the activity that arranges items or activities in order of importance relative to each other.

Systematic

The nursing process is systematic. The nurse follows specific, orderly, and logical steps based on the client's most important and often most vital needs, also known as prioritization or prioritizing. By following the logical progression of steps to identify the client's needs, the nurse can plan activities to meet them.

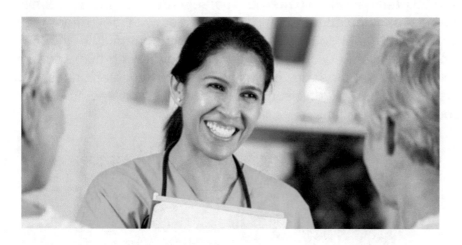

Nursing Care Plan

The Elderly Woman Hospitalized With Pneumonia

A 78-year-old woman with a history of mild heart failure treated with diuretic therapy and sodium restriction, was brought to the emergency department by her daughter. Oxygen saturation (SaO_2) via pulse oximetry is 93%. Supplemental oxygen is ordered via nasal cannula at 4 L/min. Chest x-ray reveals patchy areas of consolidation in the right middle and lower lobes. White blood cell count reveals leukocytosis (increased white blood cells). Her daughter states, "I just thought that she had a bad cold, but now she's been coughing up some thick yellow mucus and says that it is hard to breathe." A sputum culture obtained was positive for streptococcus. The client is admitted to the hospital.

KEYWORD

Leukocytosis is a condition in which the white cell (leukocyte count) is above the normal range in the blood.

Data Collection/Nursing Assessment

CThe client is diaphoretic (sweating profusely) and pale with complaints of shortness of breath. Temperature, 102.6°F (39.2°C) orally; pulse, 126 beats per minute (bpm); respirations, 38 breaths per minute, use of accessory muscles noted; blood pressure (BP), 100/60. Lungs with scattered coarse crackles (moist bubbling sounds as inhaled air comes in contact with secretions) and decreased breath sounds, especially in the right middle and lower lobes. The client describes a productive cough with thick, purulent sputum several times in the last hour. The daughter states, "I've tried to get her to drink some fluids, but she just seems so tired, coughing all the time."

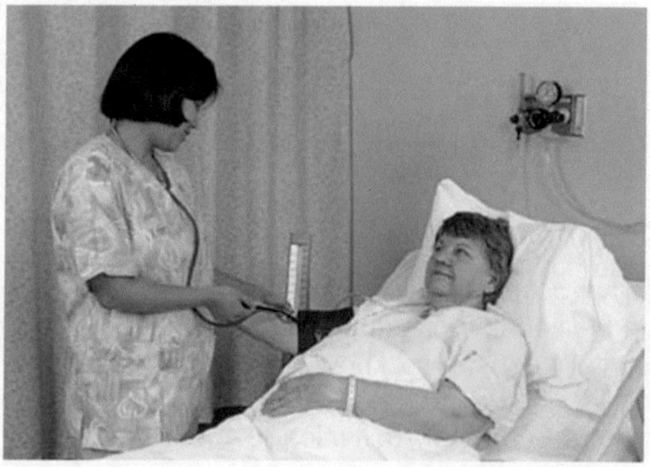

Nursing Diagnosis

Ineffective airway clearance related to physiologic effects of pneumonia as evidenced by increased sputum, coughing, abnormal breath sounds, tachypnea, and dyspnea.

KEYWORD

Arterial blood gas (ABG) test measures the oxygen and carbon dioxide levels in your blood as well your blood's pH balance.

Planning

Short-term Goals

1. Within 4–6 hours, oxygen saturation will be maintained at 95% or greater with the use of supplemental oxygen.
2. Within 24 hours, the client will state that breathing is easier.
3. By day 2 of hospitalization, the client's vital signs and arterial blood gas levels will be within expected ranges for age.

Long-term Goals

4. By discharge, the client's lungs will be clear to auscultation, and oxygen saturation will remain at greater than 95% without the use of supplemental oxygen.
5. At the time of discharge, the client and daughter will verbalize measures for continued therapy and follow-up to prevent a recurrence.

Implementation

Nursing Action

Administer supplemental, humidified oxygen via nasal cannula at the prescribed flow rate. Rationale: Supplemental, humidified oxygen aids in improving ventilation, thereby minimizing the risk for hypoxemia without drying the mucous membranes.

Nursing Action

Monitor oxygen saturation levels via pulse oximetry; assist with obtaining arterial blood gases (ABGs) as ordered. Rationale: Oxygen saturation levels and ABGs provide objective evidence of the client's tissue oxygenation.

Evaluation

SaO_2 at 95% via pulse oximetry; ABGs results confirm oxygen saturation at 95% and PaO_2 at 92 mm Hg with supplemental oxygen therapy.

Nursing Action

Assist client to assume semi-Fowler's to high Fowler's position and reposition frequently. Rationale: A position in which the client's head is elevated facilitates breathing and promotes optimal lung expansion by relieving pressure on the diaphragm. Frequent repositioning prevents pooling and stasis of secretions.

KEYWORD

Diaphragm is a thin skeletal muscle that sits at the base of the chest and separates the abdomen from the chest.

Evaluation

Decreased use of accessory muscles; client reporting a decrease in shortness of breath and decrease in difficulty breathing

Nursing Action

Assess vital signs and respiratory status, including auscultation of lung sounds, initially every 1–2 hours and then as indicated. Rationale: Frequent assessment of the client's status provides evidence of improvement or deterioration in the client's condition.

Evaluation

Temperature 100.4°F (38.0°C) orally; pulse, 100 bpm; respirations, 30 breaths per minute; BP, 110/64.

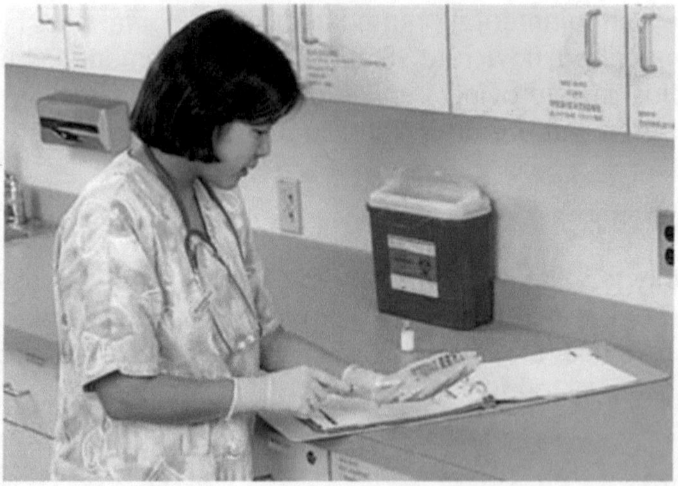

Nursing Action

Begin intravenous (IV) fluid therapy as ordered using an infusion pump; prepare antibiotic for IV infusion. Rationale: IV fluid therapy aids in replacing increased fluid lost through insensible sources and provides a route for administering IV antibiotic therapy, which is effective against the causative organism. The use of an infusion pump reduces the risk of possible fluid overload.

Client-Oriented

The nursing process is client-oriented. The needs of the client are identified, not the needs of the nurse, family, or other healthcare providers. The client and, if appropriate, the family or significant others become the nurse's partner in determining the goals for care.

A fundamental distinction between licensed nurses and nursing aides or unlicensed assistive people (UAP) is that nurses focus on the reasoning behind tasks, as opposed to merely their accomplishment. A nurse must understand when to collect vital signs, what the data reflect, and how this information relates to the client's needs, for instance. The nurse aide or UAP may know how to take vital signs, but it is not their responsibility to understand why specific actions are performed.

TIPS

As a nurse, you prioritize fulfilling the unique requirements of each patient over executing specific abilities.

Goal-Oriented

The nursing process is objective-driven. In the beginning of the nursing process, goals, objectives, and expected outcomes are set. The client, family, and important others contribute to the goal-setting process. The healthcare team guides the creation of objectives. Short-term and long-term objectives are ranked according to the client's most pressing demands and preferences. Short-term objectives are measurable outcomes that can be accomplished within hours, days, or weeks, depending on the nature of the issue. Long-term goals incorporate short-term goals, but also provide direction for the days, weeks, or months while and after a client is treated by a health professional.

Continuous

The nursing procedure is ongoing. Due to the fluctuating nature of an individual's life and health, the client's demands are often, and sometimes hourly, reassessed (or more frequently in critical care settings). Therefore, the existing nursing method must be spontaneously changed to accommodate the most current and urgent needs. The nurse must continuously reassess, set new objectives, implement new strategies, introduce new interventions, and reevaluate the whole process's performance (Figure 2.2). A nursing care plan is amended when new needs are identified, status changes occur, or it is determined that the current NCP is ineffective. Depending on the client's status, this procedure could take minutes, days, or even longer. For instance, one of the client's current goals is to get out of bed after surgery; nevertheless, the client suffers dangerously short of breath. This client requires the establishment of new objectives depending on their oxygen requirement.

Dynamic

The nursing process is dynamic and always evolving. Although there are distinct steps, they frequently overlap. Sometimes they occur simultaneously. You will acquire the capacity to utilize critical thinking abilities through experience and training. As you advance through nursing school, you will expand on the theoretical and clinical training you get at your institutions. As you create nursing care plans, you get to understand these aspects of the nursing process. Frequently, nursing care plans reflect your increased understanding of the client's demands.

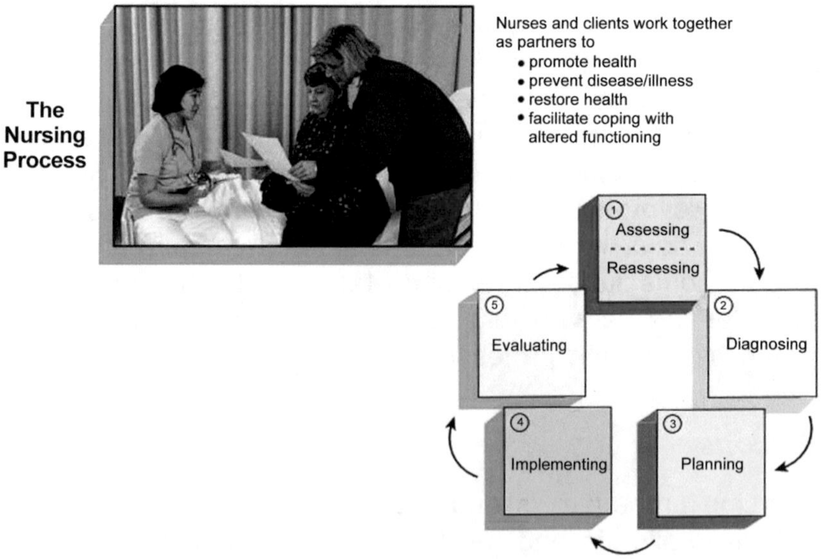

Figure 2.2: The nursing process is a continuous, scientific, systematic, client-oriented, and goal-oriented approach where the nurse and client work together to ensure quality care.

Nursing Process and Quality Care

The nursing process is a crucial instrument for providing measurable and observable evidence of the efficacy of nursing care provided in any situation. You are responsible or accountable for your activities as a registered nurse. Despite the fact that you may work with multiple customers who have the same medical issue, each individual may require unique considerations. Two of our clients, Mrs. M and Mrs. R, have recently discovered they have diabetes. Both patients must learn how to inject themselves with insulin to treat their condition. Mrs. M had no prior experience with diabetes, but Ms. R cared for her diabetic mother for several years and delivered insulin injections. Thus, you can build care plans for both clients that account for their unique educational requirements.

Care consistency is guaranteed since all nurses providing care for a patient refer to the same care plan. You can evaluate the client's progress relative to the plan. If objectives are not being accomplished, a reevaluation will reveal what additional requirements must be determined.

Remember

Nurses provide hands-on care and interventions according to the established care plan. This may include administering medications, performing treatments, assisting with activities of daily living (ADLs), monitoring vital signs, and providing emotional support.

REVIEW QUESTIONS

1. What do you understand by problem solving facility in nursing?
2. Explain about nursing process.
3. What are the steps used in the nursing process?
4. Define the characteristics of the nursing process.
5. Elaborate the nursing care plan.

MULTIPLE CHOICE QUESTIONS

1. Which part of the nursing process includes the statement of the client's actual or potential problem?

a. Nursing assessment
b. Implementation
c. Nursing diagnosis
d. Planning

2. Which of the following is a characteristic of the nursing process?

a. Instinct forms the basis for the process.
b. All health professionals use the nursing process.
c. The process occurs once for each client.
d. The client is the central focus of the process.

3. Implementation of the nursing process involves:

a. Collecting data
b. Giving actual nursing care
c. Measuring effectiveness of nursing care
d. Systematically developing goals

4. Which skill does the nurse use to determine the meaning of multiple cues when assessing clients?

a. Critical thinking
b. Evaluation
c. Experimentation
d. Nursing process

5. The primary reason for nurses to use nursing care plans is to:

a. Ensure consistency of care among all nursing staff
b. Identify client problems

c. Provide justification for nursing care
d. Utilize critical thinking skills

Answers to Multiple Choice Questions

1. (c) 2. (d) 3. (b) 4. (a) 5. (a)

REFERENCES

1. Funnell, R., Koutoukidis, G.& Lawrence, K. (2009)Tabbner's Nursing Care (5th Edition), p. 72, Elsevier Pub, Australia.
2. Ackley, B. J., &Ladwig, G. B. (2017). Nursing diagnosis handbook: An evidence-based guide to planning care (10 ed.). St. Louis: Mosby/Elsevier
3. Marriner-Tomey&Allgood (2006) Nursing Theorists and their work. p. 432
4. Reed, P. (2009) Inspired knowing in nursing. p. 63 in Loscin& Purnell (Eds) (2009) Contemporary Nursing Process.Springer Pub
5. Kim, H (2010). The Nature of Theoretical Thinking in Nursing. p. 6.
6. Bradshaw, J & Lowenstein (2010) Innovative Teaching Strategies in Nursing and Related Health Professions.
7. Funnell, R., Koutoukidis, G.& Lawrence, K. (2009) Tabbner's Nursing Care (5th Edition), p. 222, Elsevier Pub, Australia.
8. "RogerianNursingScience - Chapter 7 Practice Methods". rogeriannursingscience.wikispaces.com. Retrieved 18 April 2018.
9. Tastan, S., Linch, G. C., Keenan, G. M., Stifter, J., McKinney, D., Fahey, L., ...&Wilkie, D. J. (2014). "Evidence for the existing American Nurses Association-recognized standardized nursing terminologies: A systematic review". International Journal of Nursing Studies. 51 (8): 1160–1170. doi:10.1016/j.ijnurstu.2013.12.004. PMC 4095868. PMID 24412062.
10. Kozier, Barbara, et al. (2004) Assessing, Fundamentals of Nursing: concepts, process and practice, 2nd ed., p. 261
11. Barbara Kuhn Timby (2008-01-01), Fundamental Nursing Skills and Concepts, p. 114, ISBN 978-0-7817-7909-8

CHAPTER 3

NURSING ROLES

"A nurse is one who opens the eyes of a newborn and gently closes the eyes of a dying man. It is indeed a high blessing to be the first and last to witness the beginning and end of life."

—Unknown

INTRODUCTION

Changes in health technology, professional knowledge, skills, patient demands, and expectations have made health care a dynamic field in which to work in recent years. The aging population, the rise in chronic diseases, the development of day surgery, the expansion of primary care, and the ongoing reduction in hospital stay length have all contributed to shifting patterns of need and demand. These changes are taking place in healthcare systems all around the world, and they have an impact on the type of care offered as well as the format in which it is delivered. Such changes, in particular, have forced the establishment of new professional roles and practices. The shortage of medical doctors in health care was a particularly significant cause, prompting consideration of three major solutions: train and employ more doctors; train and employ doctor's assistants; or urge nurses to take on more medical tasks. The latter was the cheapest and quickest choice, and by the early twenty-first century, nurses were taking on more and more activities that were formerly the sole responsibility of physicians. This technique provided a significant impetus in the development of advanced practice nursing roles, which is seen as a critical issue in contemporary nursing. To address some of the challenges stated, the International Council of Nurses has identified the

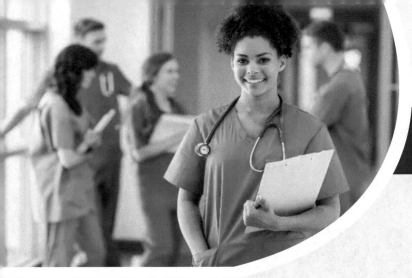

need for worldwide networking and support. There is an acknowledgment that more work needs to be done to guarantee uniformity in how these jobs are described, as well as a shared understanding of how persons should be trained for these responsibilities. It is obvious that new nursing roles exist and will continue to emerge, and we must consider whether existing nursing theories are applicable to these new roles or whether other theories may be more applicable.

LEARNING OBJECTIVES

After completing the chapter, you will be able to accomplish the following:

- Define the roles of a nurse
- Explain the role of nurses in modern healthcare
- Describe the new roles in nursing
- List some implications of the new nursing roles
- Using theory to understand new roles in nursing
- Elaborate the influence of the biomedical model on nursing roles

Key-terms

- Dignity
- Mini doctors
- Maxi nurses
- Patient satisfaction
- Physician
- Psychology
- Role theory
- Role stress
- Role strain
- Biomedical model

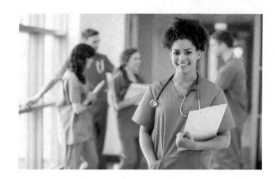

ROLES OF A NURSE

The primary role of a nurse is to advocate and care for individuals and support them through health and illness. However, there are various other responsibilities of a nurse that form a part of the role of a nurse, including to:

- Record medical history and symptoms
- Collaborate with teams to plan for patient care
- Advocate for the health and wellbeing of patients
- Monitor patient health and record signs
- Administer medications and treatments
- Operate medical equipment
- Perform diagnostic tests
- Educate patients about management of illnesses
- Provide support and advice to patients

KEYWORD

Caregiver is a paid or unpaid member of a person's social network who helps them with activities of daily living.

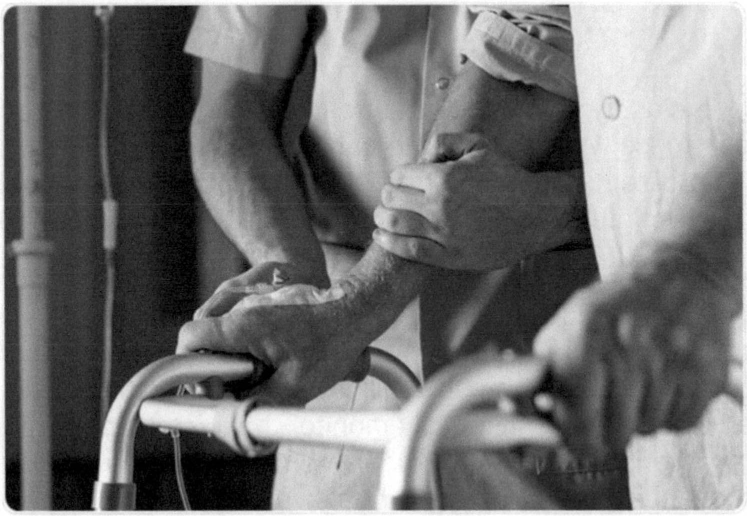

Patient Care

A nurse is a patient's caregiver who assists in the management of physical needs, the prevention of illness, and the treatment of health disorders. To accomplish this, they must examine and monitor the patient while also documenting any pertinent information to aid in treatment decision-making.

Throughout the treatment process, the nurse monitors the patient's progress and works in the best interests of the patient.

A nurse's care goes beyond the provision of drugs and other interventions. They are in charge of patients' holistic treatment, which includes their emotional, developmental, cultural, and spiritual needs.

Patient Advocacy

The nurse's main priority is the patient. The nurse's responsibility is to advocate for the patient's best interests and to safeguard the patient's dignity during treatment and care. This may entail making recommendations in patients' treatment plans in consultation with other health experts.

This is especially crucial because people who are ill are frequently unable to comprehend medical circumstances and respond normally. The nurse's responsibility is to always support the patient and represent the patient's best interests, especially while treatment decisions are being made.

KEYWORD

Medical team refers to a group of healthcare professionals who work together to provide comprehensive and coordinated care to patients.

Planning of Care

A nurse is closely involved in the treatment of a patient's decision-making process. When analyzing patient indicators and recognizing potential problems, they must be able to think critically in order to make appropriate recommendations and actions.

Because other health professionals, such as doctors or specialists, are usually in charge of making final treatment decisions, nurses must be able to properly communicate facts about patient health. Nurses are the most familiar with each particular patient's situation since they continuously monitor their signs and symptoms, and they should interact with other members of the medical team to promote the greatest patient health outcomes.

Patient Education and Support

Nurses must also ensure that patients understand their health, ailments, drugs, and treatments to the best of their abilities. This is critical when patients are discharged from the hospital and must manage their own treatments.

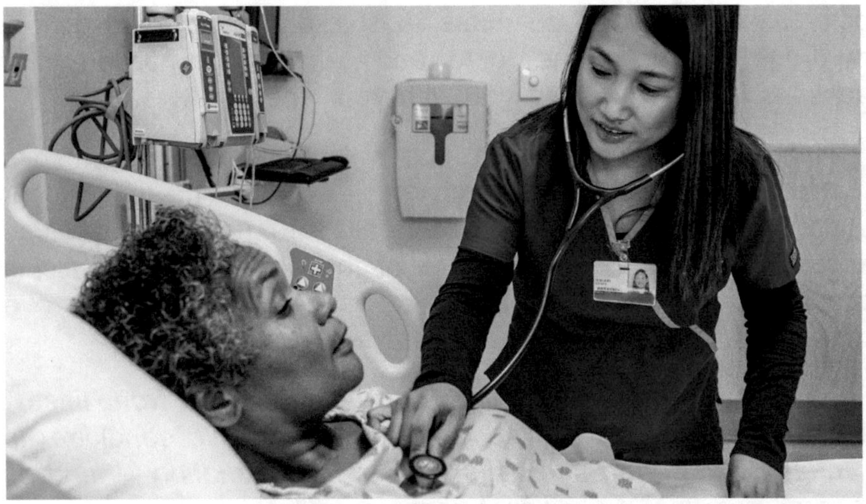

KEYWORD

Medical community means the physicians and allied healthcare specialists located and available within a definable geographic area.

THE ROLE OF NURSES IN MODERN HEALTHCARE

Nurses have historically provided the general public with high-quality treatment. Professional respect in the medical community, on the other hand, was earned via years of lobbying, organization, and, most significantly, intellectual advancement of the profession. Nurses were viewed as less integral members of a clinical care team 70 years ago (despite their many responsibilities), but they have fought for more recognition and now command much more respect and autonomy, enjoying an increasingly collaborative relationship with physicians and other healthcare professionals.

To understand why nurses are so vital in healthcare today, consider what registered nurses perform, from the relationships they build with patients to how they collaborate with other practitioners.

Nurses Spend More Time with Patients

Consider a recent doctor's appointment. A nurse was most likely the first person you saw after checking in at the front desk. He or she most likely made a small conversation while asking about your health and checking your vitals. That small conversation, on the other hand, wasn't only to put you at ease or to avoid silence.

Skilled nurses understand that spending time getting to know patients can be incredibly beneficial in unearthing critical health information that patients might not reveal otherwise. After the doctor examined you, the nurse most likely returned to go over any drugs ordered by the doctor and to ask if you had any more questions before assisting you with your check-out.

Nurses spend even more time with patients in the hospital. In a recently published research article, of the time critical care patients spent with at least one healthcare practitioner, nurses accounted for approximately 86% of that time, while physicians accounted for only 13%. The time spent with nurses was even greater during overnight hospital stays.

Nurses are often described as serving on the front lines of healthcare — the first to notice when a patient's condition has changed or to spring into action in a critical situation — and this research certainly makes that case.

KEYWORD

Healthcare practitioner is a professional who provides medical or healthcare services to individuals, families, and communities. These practitioners are trained and licensed in their respective fields to diagnose, treat, and manage various health conditions.

Nurses as Patient Advocates

The time nurses spend with patients provides them with a unique understanding of their patients' wants and requirements, behaviors, health habits, and worries, so making them crucial advocates in their treatment. In fact, the American Nurses Association identifies advocacy as a "pillar of nursing" and considers it to be one of the most fundamental reasons why nurses are essential to healthcare.

A nurse's advocacy role can also take numerous forms. During a conversation with a patient's family member, for instance, a nurse may discover a vital element that is not recorded in the patient's medical records and transmit this information to the healthcare team. Or, if a nurse is concerned that a medicine is not functioning as expected, she may contact the pharmacist to discuss the issue.

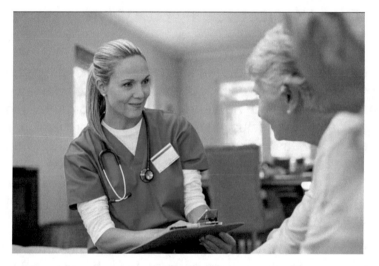

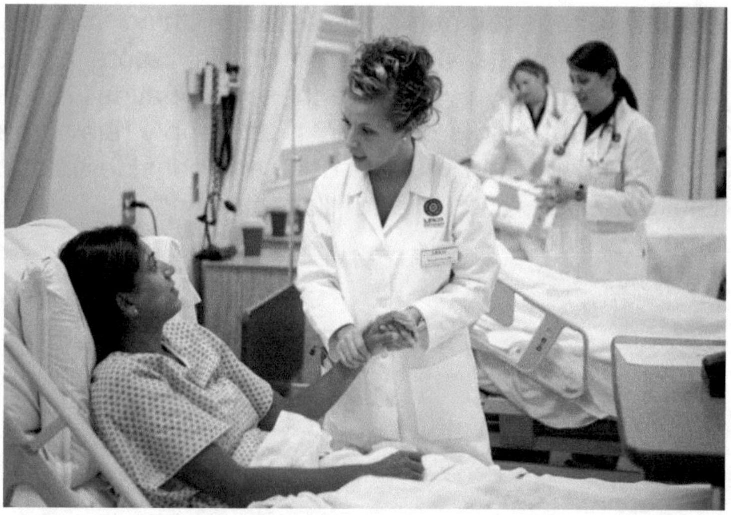

Education as a Critical Function of Nursing

A challenge felt across the U.S. healthcare industry is low health literacy among healthcare populations. Health literacy is the capacity to comprehend fundamental health facts in order to make educated decisions.

Deep scientific knowledge of the field of medicine, which is one of the factors that makes doctors so effective at their jobs, can be difficult to convey when discussing sophisticated medical terminology with patients. In addition, some people may feel intimidated by the medical community or lack the knowledge to ask the appropriate questions.

A significant portion of nurses' time and energy is devoted to teaching patients. This may be helping them understand a therapy or process, outlining drugs and side effects, highlighting the significance of healthy nutrition and excellent hygiene, or describing how a clinic functions (in the case of ongoing treatment).

TIPS

Assisting in the coordination of a patient's care with another provider's office or ensuring that a patient has been granted informed permission prior to a procedure may also constitute patient advocacy.

Nurses and their Role in Monitoring Patients' Health

The function of nurses in today's complicated healthcare environment cannot be discussed without including the monitoring of patient care and maintenance of records. Previously, we examined the position of nurses at the forefront of patient care. Although physicians and other members of the care team also check on patients, nurses are responsible for daily monitoring of their condition.

In assessing patients, nurses record everything from their vital signs and reason for the visit to their fall risk score and current prescriptions. Then, they synthesize these evaluations, update the permanent medical records of patients, and apply relevant fees (a function of billing). In fact, nurses devote a considerable amount of effort to updating records and disseminating vital information to the larger care team.

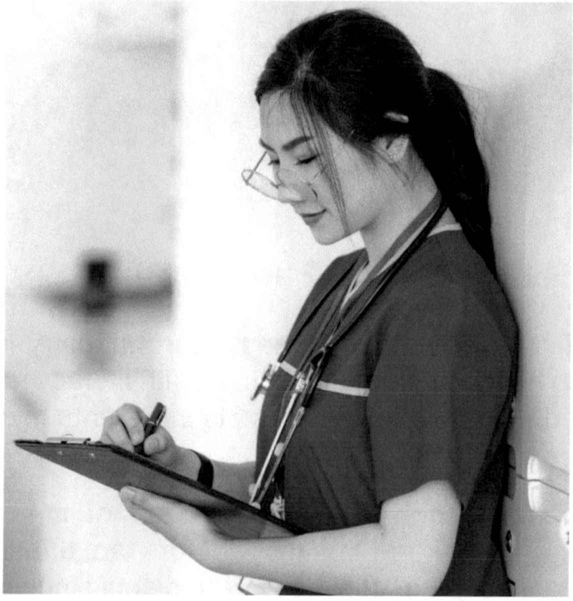

Did you Know?

In the United States, 19.2% of nursing positions are held by people of minority backgrounds. The remaining 80.8% of positions are held by Caucasian individuals, particularly women. Diversity in nursing is lacking. Low numbers of diverse populations in the nursing field can create difficulties in treating diverse patients.

Nurses Today Have Greater Autonomy Than You Might Think

Having read about the nursing profession, you are likely aware that nurses now have more autonomy than in the past. What does this precisely mean? In the case of hospital stays in particular, nurses are frequently the first to identify a problem, and while contacting the attending physician is standard procedure, there are occasions when nurses must act promptly to stabilize the patient.

In other instances, as part of the order set, a physician may specify situations in which a nurse may act without the doctor's authorization. (For instance, if a patient's magnesium levels fall below a certain threshold, the nurse may administer magnesium without consulting the physician.)

NEW ROLES IN NURSING

Internationally, the majority of nations provide some form of nursing foundation training, upon completion of which a person is considered to have attained the status of a nurse. In the United Kingdom, for instance, a newly qualified individual is permitted to register as a nurse and will have earned either a bachelor's degree or a diploma. The structure of nursing professions in the United Kingdom can be depicted as a "practice cross" in which the freshly certified nurse is viewed as a novice who can advance to become a practitioner with more expertise. On initial registration, they are also considered generalists as opposed to specialists, however, they may advance to more specialized responsibilities.

KEYWORD

Standardization is the process of developing, promoting and possibly mandating standards-based and compatible technologies and processes within an industry.

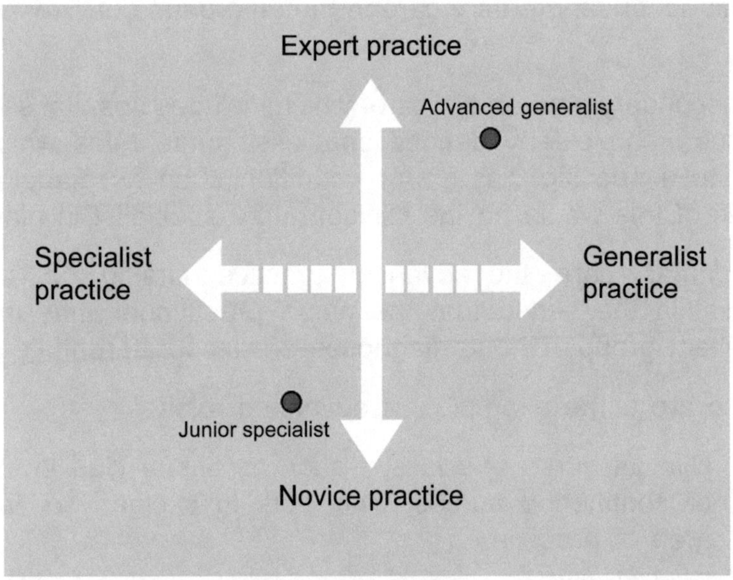

In tracing the evolution of specialized positions, it was discovered that clinical nurse specialists were first established in the United States, where the extended traditional nursing function did not threaten the interaction between nursing and medicine. In the subsequent evolution, the nurse practitioner role, nurses expanded their scope of practice to include diagnosis. Later in the chapter, the distinctions between role expansion and extension will be discussed. This prompted great debate over whether nurse practitioners are "maxi nurses" or "mini doctors." In the United States, these responsibilities grew and evolved until it became apparent that there was a need for standardization of practice and education requirements. In the UK, a trend resembling that in the United States arose. In particular, Barbara Stilwell's work as a nurse practitioner in primary care in the 1980s was regarded as a turning point in the evolution of advanced nursing professions. As in the United States, the growth of advanced nursing roles in the 1990s in the United Kingdom was marked by a lack of a defined clinical career structure, conflicts over the purpose and scope of such practitioners, and a lack of consensus regarding an approved degree of educational preparation. This resulted in a multiplicity of titles and varied sorts of preparation (or, in some cases, none at all) and was affected by the health service's short-term needs. In the United Kingdom, the demand for these new roles within the National Health Service continues to rise, but their development has been hampered by variance in role names and preparation, as well as concerns regarding competence and governance. In the United Kingdom, there appear to be distinctions between primary care and secondary/tertiary care in the emergence of new nursing jobs.

KEYWORD

Medical intervention means the ability to assess the situation and contact the appropriate medical professional, not the direct application of medical care.

In secondary and tertiary care, which includes hospital settings, the focus is on clearly defined specialist nurse roles which are related to a specific disease or condition such as diabetes. An example of this would be the clinical nurse specialist in diabetes.

In primary care, the advanced practice nursing job is more generalist in the sense that the nurse practitioner may interact with patient groups whose diagnoses are less differentiated.

Here are some examples of advanced roles:

- Clinical nurse specialists, such as tissue viability nurses or continence nurses, who work in a clearly delineated area of practice.
- Public health nurses, who operate in specialized community roles, and nurse practitioners, who can diagnose, provide therapies (including medications), and manage units with minimal medical intervention.
- Consultant nurses.

The situation was unclear, and the lack of consistency meant that there was no consensus regarding the preparation of these practitioners, how their role would be judged, or whether it could be transferred to other fields. Inconsistencies in role growth and a conflict between personal and professional ideals were also caused by local policies. Additionally, there were geographical differences in the number and type of specialized nurses, notably in isolated and rural areas.

In this context, there was much discussion regarding the modernization of nursing careers, strategic workforce planning (the need for a flexible, well-educated, and competent workforce), and the lack of clarity around advanced practice responsibilities. In the United Kingdom, the Scottish Government's development of the Advanced Practice Toolkit and the "practice cross" was highly significant. In addition, work was performed to clarify and distinguish expert and advanced practice.

- Specialist practice is viewed as a specialized, context-specific function, such as that of a tissue viability nurse.
- Advanced practice is a level of practice, not a function, and is not limited to the clinical domain; it also includes people who work in research, education, or managerial/ leadership and are capable of making high-level judgments.

Remember

Nurses are the most familiar with the individual patient situation as they monitor their signs and symptoms on an ongoing basis and should collaborate with other members of the medical team to promote the best patient health outcomes.

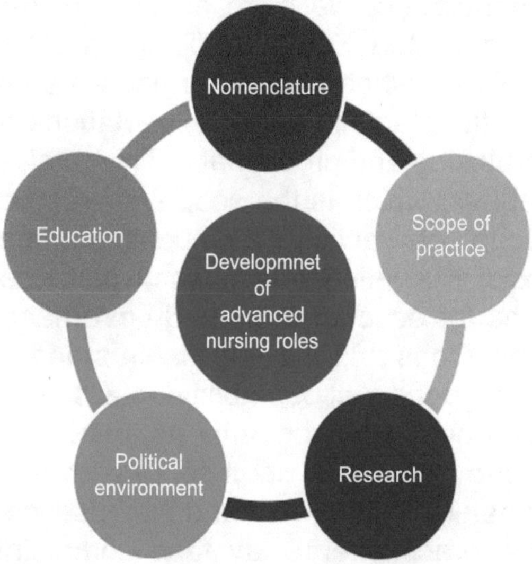

Figure 3.1: Development of advanced nursing roles.

The Advanced Practice Toolkit also identified that advanced practice should be founded on four pillars: clinical, research, education and management/ leadership. These four pillars, it was suggested, should underpin the work of advanced practice nurses regardless of their particular role.

SOME IMPLICATIONS OF THE NEW NURSING ROLES

The development of these advanced practice roles in nursing, as we have seen, has not been unproblematic and was characterized by inconsistency in role development, in titles and in how individuals might be prepared for these roles. We have taken the UK as an example to illustrate these issues, but these concerns were not confined to the UK. Figure 3.1 identified and explored five main issues pertinent to the development of advanced practice nursing roles internationally:

- Nomenclature
- Scope of practice and prescriptive authority
- Education for these roles
- Political environment
- Research into role outcome.

KEYWORD

Accountability in the workplace can mean that all employees are accountable for their own actions, behaviors, performance and decisions.

Nomenclature and Scope of Practice

In terms of nomenclature, we have alluded to the multiplicity of terms used in the United Kingdom. There are thirteen different titles internationally for what may be termed an advanced practice function. Different titles entail varying expectations of role conduct, which can be perplexing and problematic. This relates to the second fundamental problem, which is the scope of practice and power to prescribe. The scope of practice encompassed numerous activities, including diagnosis, evaluation, and, in some instances, prescription. This has concerns for accountability and governance because the extent of these new jobs and the applicable standards of behavior are frequently ambiguous. Accountability entails accepting personal responsibility for one's conduct, and no individual can be held accountable for the actions of another. Due to the inventive and ground-breaking nature of their work and the absence of clear advice on accountability, practitioners may face complaints, disciplinary action, or legal action if something goes wrong.

The challenges surrounding the accountability and duty assumed by those in inventive roles have included discussions on the application of theories, protocols, and protocols. If the function is truly innovative, then tight adherence to outdated notions could inhibit innovation. The same holds true for the possible protective effect of evidence-based protocols, which are viewed by some as being too restrictive. In the United Kingdom, theories, guidelines, and protocols do not carry the power of legislative regulation; hence, there is a discussion as to whether a new section of the UK Nursing and Midwifery Council register for advanced practice nurses is necessary. According to the current situation (which may change), there is no need for a new part to be added to the register. This is not the case in other nations where nurse practitioners are subject to different requirements and licenses than those required for initial registration.

KEYWORD

Medical territory could range from a local community clinic serving a specific neighborhood to healthcare systems that cover a larger region or even international medical teams providing care in underserved areas.

Education, Political Environment and Research

The third noted difficulty was the requisite education for these new professions. Seventy-one percent of the 31 nations surveyed had formal education programs to educate practitioners for advanced practice responsibilities.

In addition, they emphasized the significance of the health care environment and the political forces that facilitated the creation of advanced practice practitioners. As previously noted, this was a response to health care demands and a physician shortage in some areas of primary care in the United States. High percentages of advanced nurse practitioners working in secondary and tertiary care were discovered in a survey, showing a strong tendency toward specialist practice. Finally, they highlighted the ongoing necessity for studies on patient outcomes following treatment by advanced practitioners. They did acknowledge that research findings in this area suggest good outcomes and levels of patient satisfaction for those receiving care from advanced practice nurses.

USING THEORY TO UNDERSTAND NEW ROLES IN NURSING

We emphasized the significance of theory and the various levels of nursing-appropriate theory in terms of sophistication and abstraction. In this section, we revisit the contribution of theory to comprehending the evolution and influence of these new nursing positions. Any conversation concerning the growth of advanced nursing practice must include, for instance, the boundaries between medical and nursing practice and the duties of both doctors and nurses, particularly as nurses expand their activities into what may be considered conventional medical territory. In order to comprehend the contribution of theory to advanced practice nursing, we will examine role theory, the impact and influence of the biological model, and if nursing theories have anything to contribute to these new nursing roles.

Role Theory

KEYWORD

Amoeba is a type of cell or unicellular organism with the ability to alter its shape, primarily by extending and retracting pseudopods.

It is essential to comprehend role theory in the context of emerging nursing role innovations. This tendency has been described using two terms: role expansion and role extension. The former entails that nurses maintain their occupational concentration while assuming a broader responsibility. For instance, if a nurse's position centered on health promotion, expanding their participation in health promotion would be an example of role expansion. In contrast, role extension happens when nurses expand their responsibilities into another discipline in an almost amoeba-like manner. Thus, for nurses to assume prescription responsibilities or do minor surgical procedures would constitute a role expansion. This increases the likelihood of position ambiguity, role overlap, and role conflict. These arise at the point where doctors are relinquishing responsibilities that were once solely their responsibility and nurses are assuming these responsibilities. Unless both parties arrive at the same conclusion at the same time, role conflict and uncertainty may result. Care quality and patient safety may be compromised in such situations.

Using a Sociological Perspective on Role

In the social sciences, specifically sociology and psychology, theories regarding roles can be found. Using sociological theories, it is possible to identify different ways of thinking about roles, which fall into two broad categories of social thought. The first is structural functionalism, which holds that the successful fulfillment of duties is essential to the social system's stability. An important thinker, Talcott Parsons, presented the concept of the "sick role" as an illustration. In contrast to the biological model, which views sickness as a 'biomedical, mechanical breakdown,' Parsons viewed illness as a 'deviation from social standards' that required medical approval. In a situation involving illness, therefore, both the doctor and the patient have roles, and with these positions come rights and responsibilities. These rights and responsibilities assist to create expectations for how both parties, patient and physician, should conduct their respective duties.

Another expansive viewpoint is that of 'agency,' in which individuals as social agents have autonomy and the ability to alter their environment. In this view, individuals play a role in how they show themselves in the social sphere. The metaphor of a theater in which individuals act out their roles according to the scenario or setting in which they are placed. To meet the expectations that others may have of the nurse's function, the nurse will take a specific role and conduct herself in a particular manner when caring for patients. Consider this to be "front-stage" behavior, i.e., the behavior that satisfies the expectations of others in that environment. However, Goffman also discussed "backstage" conduct. Here, away from patients' view, nurses may behave in ways that may or may not appear compatible with their behaviors onstage.

KEYWORD

Social position is the position of an individual in a given society and culture. A given position may belong to many individuals.

The concept of role can be explained by various theories. These are not nursing theories, but they can be used in nursing in an effort to comprehend important role-related concerns and how they may affect nursing. The introduction of advanced nurse practitioners resulted in a shift in the duties of both the individuals engaged and the nursing profession as a whole. The pioneering nurse practitioners were learning expertise and expanding their practice into the medical area as they altered their roles. Using such theories within these sociological perspectives enables us to comprehend the role that roles play in complicated social systems such as health care. As a result of a certain role, certain behaviors and practices are expected. Therefore, it is extremely unsettling when people or occupational groups, such as nurses, fail to correspond to these standards. Role theory is a collection of notions and propositions in the form of hypothetical predictions of how people would perform in a specific occupation or under what conditions certain sorts of behavior might be anticipated. The expectations of how people should behave in a certain social position are crucial to this. Concepts within role theory include:

- role norms
- role set
- role stress
- role confusion
- role overlap
- role conflict.

Role norms and Role Sets

In considering roles, the structural functionalist perspective remains relevant. In the minds of members of a group, 'role norms' outline what they should do and what is expected of them under particular situations. There are also role expectations held by members of the individual's "role set" that impose pressure on the individual's performance in a specific setting. The 'role set' refers to the role relationships maintained by virtue of a specific social standing. For instance, a nurse's 'role set' would normally include nursing colleagues, other health professional colleagues, patients, and organization representatives.

KEYWORD

Nursing practice involves advocacy for the rights of the individual patient and for their family.

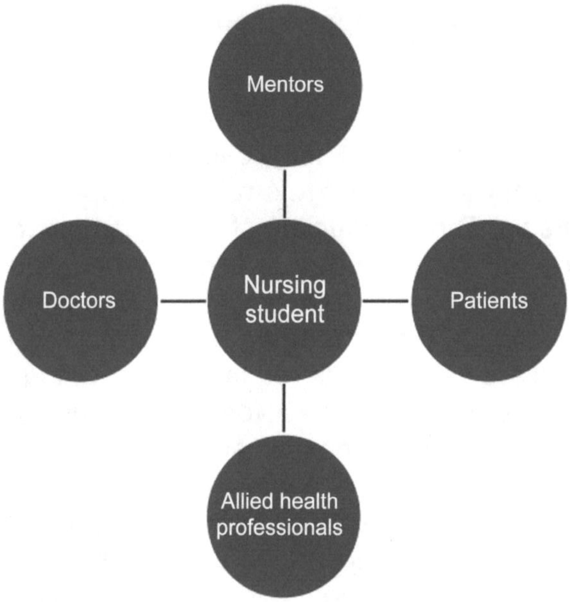

Figure 3.2: Role sets.

The consideration of role is of particular relevance to those involved in new roles in nursing. After all, the context in which they work is changing and therefore the perceptions and expectations of their role are also changing.

Role Stress and Strain

'Role stress and role strain' in nursing as related to the work environment. A workplace with high job demands, minimal assistance from colleagues, and a lack of key resources makes it extremely difficult for employees to fulfill their role responsibilities, resulting in role strain. There is evidence that the introduction of additional nursing jobs has resulted in instances of role-related stress and strain for the nurses engaged.

The boundaries between inter- and intra-professional practices and competencies were blurring as the nursing practice became more diversified. Consequently, due to the ambiguity around role development and professional isolation, there is a risk for 'role stress' among those who occupy new nursing responsibilities. Innovative jobs can lead to isolation, 'burnout,' and role dissonance, particularly when the organization provides no support. Managerial support is seen as a crucial aspect of a smooth transfer to new jobs.

The innovative nature of some positions can also make it difficult to communicate with colleagues in comparable positions. This indicates that there are little possibilities to discuss professional and practice difficulties and identify potential mentors. Furthermore, coworkers may fail to recognize the skills and value of the incumbent. For personal and professional identification, as well as for offering a resource for support and debriefing, it was essential to form ties with coworkers who had similar positions and theoretical ideas. Moreover, if various advanced practitioners utilize different ideas to inform their practice, this could foster isolation and prevent the sharing of best practices.

Role Conflict

Role conflict is described as divergence between the role expectations of various role set members. Bower et al. (2004) examined the introduction of a new primary health care role and concluded that the requirements for the post-holder in the new role and the existing staff's expectations increased the likelihood of role conflict. Professional and lay perspectives on generic and specialist responsibilities in the community were discussed, and it was highlighted that there was apprehension that specialization (although desirable) might result in role conflict, role overlap, and role confusion. A method of action research to investigate the effects of one new function (interprofessional care coordinators) in a big London trust. They observed that the conflicts resulting from this new position were due to the position's incompatibility with the hospital's established hierarchy. Evaluation of a cancer nurse specialist function revealed the same lack of compatibility with existing systems. In the latter instance, the nurse's emphasis on compassion and care was in contradiction with the physician's concentration on technology and treatment. Multiple factors have led to the pervasiveness of role ambiguity and conflict in nursing. Redefining role boundaries has never been more vital than it is today, he concluded, despite the fact that the contribution of nursing is difficult to identify in an expanding profession.

Remember

A nurse should take the time to explain to the patient and their family or caregiver what to do and what to expect when they leave the hospital or medical clinic.

THE INFLUENCE OF THE BIOMEDICAL MODEL ON NURSING ROLES

Previously, we examined sociological role theories to assist us comprehend how ideas from a different academic field, such as sociology, might lead to a better understanding of the nursing function within health care systems. In this section, we examine a medical paradigm, the biomedical model, which nurses may employ in their new advanced practice positions. The biomedical model consists of assessment, diagnosis, prescription, and treatment, to put it simply. It is the theoretical framework utilized by the majority of physicians in their daily practice. The evolution of advanced and specialized responsibilities has had repercussions for the education and preparation of nurses for these positions. Certain professions need nurses to acquire advanced assessment, diagnostics, and prescribing abilities, which have historically been the exclusive purview of medical practice. Therefore, the educational provision for these nurses had to include the necessary knowledge and abilities for performing these responsibilities.

KEYWORD

Physicians is a person qualified to practice medicine, especially one who specializes in diagnosis and medical treatment as distinct from surgery.

A Brief History of the Biomedical Model

The biological paradigm has a lengthy history, thus it should come as no surprise that it has affected the development of some nursing ideas and nursing duties while hindering the development of others. Florence Nightingale (1859) believed that the functions of medicine and nursing should be properly differentiated. Prior to the founding of her nurse training program at St. Thomas's Hospital in London, nurses resembled SaireyGamp in their lowly status. In contrast, physicians hailed from the respectable middle and upper middle classes, and their social and educational backgrounds were generally vastly apart from those of their subordinate nurses. Therefore, in the 19th century of Florence Nightingale, doctors and nurses were differentiated by gender, social status, language, and education, a distinction that lasted for the majority of the 20th century.

The biomedical model's scientific foundation can be traced back to Hippocrates, Aristotle, and Galen. Descartes promoted the concept of the body as a machine in the early seventeenth century. Disease was considered as the result of machine failure, and the physician's job was to fix the equipment. This essential concept of reductionism underpins the treatment philosophy of the majority of medical professionals. This suggests that all behavioral phenomena must be conceptualized using physiochemical concepts. This fundamental principle has been recognized over the years not just by many health care professionals but also by the general population.

The Biomedical Model Process

Within the biomedical model, the importance of the initial evaluation to physicians cannot be overstated. The initial examination will eventually lead to the identification of symptoms. To confirm the presence of sickness, proponents of the biological model have a vested interest in seeking anomalous clinical characteristics. These indications and symptoms are classified into patterns that serve as the foundation for diagnostic labeling. Because the client is viewed as little more than a sickness entity, such labeling has a dehumanizing effect.

According to the biomedical model, knowledge of the condition defines the therapeutic approach. However, the goals of therapy may not be client-centered, and the individual may assume the roles of patient and client with the need to participate. This cooperation is a crucial component of the therapeutic procedure.

Historically, nurses were also expected to comply with and cooperate with physician directions. Therefore, despite the fact that the therapy plan may give the appearance of an egalitarian team approach, the doctor was seen as superior to all other health professionals.

KEYWORD

Diagnostic labeling of mood disorders can lead to more bleak assessments from hypothetical colleagues according to one study, though its impact on desire for social distance was rather mixed

Benefits of the Biomedical Model

The biomedical model has significant benefits for the treatment of disease. Many clients have been liberated from distressing symptomatology as a result of advances in medically oriented treatments, which has led to their early discharge. The public finds it reassuring to be cared for inside a framework they are familiar with since it is familiar to prospective clients. These elements and the contribution of the biological model must be understood by nurses in new roles. Nevertheless, nursing's dissatisfaction with the biological model's pervasiveness has been one of the primary causes for the formation of nursing theories. The biomedical approach is no longer sufficient now that nurses add their unique perspective to the work.

Limitations of the Biomedical Model

KEYWORD

Substitution is a type of mutation in which one nucleotide is replaced by a different nucleotide.

The limits of the biological paradigm for nursing quickly became apparent as a result of the intense scrutiny by nurse theorists and experts from other fields. In the conventional health care system, nurses held a submissive position as handmaidens. Many attributed this subservient position to a stubborn reliance on the biological model.

Nurses, frequently authored by physicians, clergy, or psychologists, reminded nurses that theory was too difficult for them and that they did not need to think, but rather to just follow regulations, be obedient, be compassionate, perform their duty, and carry out medical directives.

As an observer of signs and symptoms, the nurse was the doctor's eyes and ears; as a practitioner, he or she was the doctor's hands and feet, administering the prescribed therapy. There was a risk that nurses would disregard client characteristics that did not cleanly fit within the limitations of the biological model if they were limited to a particular duty. Constrained by this model, nurses were ill-equipped to care for the complete patient and family. The nursing profession's devotion to physicians' directives developed a fixation on cure, with caring frequently taking second place. It is hardly surprising that, when confronted with illness, the public places a premium on treatment. However, treatment without care is a meaningless phenomenon, and many chronic and terminal illnesses require a focus on care and palliation rather than treatment.

The Biomedical Model and New Roles in Nursing

Given the limitations of the biomedical model, there has been concern about the emergence of new nursing positions in traditionally medically-managed domains. One of the ways these roles were developed was through medical substitution, in which nurses took on roles and responsibilities formerly associated with medicine. This change is appealing to the nursing profession, which has been plagued by insecurity, poor status, and gender inequity. However, there is a risk of nursing specialists adopting a medicalized work description. This is partially due to the inability of the nursing profession to define both specialized and general nursing practice. Those questioning the function of the specialty nurse and nurse practitioner have also cited the potential de-skilling of the "generalist" nurse as a worry. Intriguingly, specialized nurses may wish to keep their specialized expertise to themselves, while generalist nurses may be content to leave difficult patient care issues to their specialized peers.

The possible de-skilling of clinical nurses will be raised by nursing students. This was due to the generalist allegedly "passing the buck" to the specialist and the specialist allegedly adopting a superiority complex over the generalist. It is also likely that the most skilled and qualified nurses are "creamed off" to specialized roles, which could be detrimental to the remaining personnel and possibly result in a decline in results and standards.

It is a given that, as a result of new technologies, knowledge, and skills, all professions advance to new practices, leaving behind what may be viewed as dull jobs and responsibilities. Ultimately, to remain professionally stagnant is to regress. Recognizing this, nurses must be cautious about what they remove from their professional portfolios. If they embark on more medical work without consideration, they risk becoming little more than technicians and transferring to unqualified assistants the practices that patients and their families value most. If nurses were to become "mini-doctors," would they have a greater affinity for the biological model, or would they carry the best of nursing theory with them?

KEYWORD

Meta-theory is a theory whose subject matter is theory itself, aiming to describe existing theory in a systematic way.

The Relevance of Existing Nursing Theory to New Nursing Roles

There are three principal levels of theory, with meta-theory frequently considered a fourth level. In this section, however, we will concentrate on the three levels that somewhat resemble the classifications of grand theory, mid-range theory, and practical theory. It will be claimed that big theory is of limited use to nurses who have assumed additional responsibilities. For these nurses, the less abstract and more easily operationalizable mid-range and practice theories have become critical.

Relevance of Existing 'Grand' Nursing Theories

There were over 50 nursing theories, most of which were formulated many decades ago. The obvious point to consider is whether these old theories are still relevant to the new roles that nurses are undertaking or whether there is a need for their adaptation or their amalgamation with the biomedical model.

Needs	Interaction	Outcome	Caring/becoming
• Henderson (1966) • Orem (1959) • Roper et al. (1983) • Abdellah (1960)	• Peplau (1952) • King (1968) • Johnson (1959) • Orlando (1961) • Travelbee (1966) • Paterson & Zderad (1976)	• Levine (1966) • Roy (1970) • Neuman (1972) • Rogers (1970)	• Newman (1976) • Watson (1979) • Leininger (1978) • Parse (1981)

Figure 3.3: Classification and examples of nursing 'grand' theories.

Limitations of 'Grand' Theories

The majority of nursing's grand theories have been tried but not tested. Many nurses were dissatisfied with their expansive breadth and lack of clarity. While the philosophical foundations of self-care, interpersonal relationships, adaptation, and interaction are still important for nurses, their inability to be operationalized has been a source of frustration, and their use as frameworks to develop and guide practice has declined in the late 20th and early 21st centuries.

Using a 21st-century lens, it is possible to claim that great ideas were developed for a different age and a different type of nurse. In the same way that nurse educators frequently chastise nursing students for reading out-of-date literature, we should examine whether utilizing nursing theories written forty or fifty years ago is still appropriate, given that nursing has evolved philosophically and practically. It may be claimed that new theories are required to account for the numerous new roles that nurses are assuming. Even while nursing has expanded into medicine, the biological paradigm will not serve nurses well in the brave new world of advanced and specialty practice.

Relevance of Existing 'Mid-range' Nursing Theories

For practice disciplines, middle-range theories were especially vital. This is extremely relevant to the creation of new positions. Specialist and advanced nurses require research-based ideas that may be used for the delivery and improvement of patient care. Over two decades ago, there was a need for the creation of mid-range ideas regarding the treatment of pain and the promotion of sleep, despite the fact that these topics have only recently received increased attention in the United Kingdom. The moment is ripe for nurses to create and utilize mid-range theories in their new jobs.

There are numerous theories with the potential for straightforward application in practice. Some, such as Orem's mid-range theory of self-care deficiency, came from "grand" theories, while others emerged inductively from practice. The example we provided was Swanson's (1991) mid-range theory for application in perinatal nursing, and the scenario was miscarriage. There are further moderate hypotheses about menstrual care, family caregiving, relapse among ex-smokers, and ambiguity in sickness, the peri-menopausal phase, self-transcendence, personal risk-taking, and illness trajectory. The elegance of mid-range theories is that they are easily applicable to practice. It has been emphasized in the preceding discussion that new nurses are frequently professionally isolated. Mid-range theories can offer them with the theoretical and professional assurance required for autonomy and accountability in their new responsibilities. Nonetheless, it is essential to recognize the threat they offer to communication and collaboration between generalist and specialist nurses, as well as across specialties.

Remember

Knowledge brokers facilitate the transfer and exchange of knowledge from where it is abundant to where it is needed, thereby supporting co-development and improving the innovative capability of organizations in their network.

The Place of Theory in Advanced Practice Education

Initially, some advanced practice and specialist responsibilities were formed and granted to postholders who had amassed a vast amount of expertise through prolonged immersion in clinical settings. Subsequently, there were calls for advanced practitioners to be educated to at least the master's level and to be taught specialized skills and information pertinent to their new position. Advanced practitioners are expected to have enough levels of 'know how' knowledge, which is supplemented by 'know that' knowledge taught in Master's studies. What kind of "know that" knowledge should be taught in these programs is an important question. As stated in prior chapters, the knowledge utilized in nursing practice is complicated and diverse. Advanced practice nurses lay a strong emphasis on following evidence-based guidelines. This is reflective of the present health care environment, which prioritizes evidence-based practice and places special emphasis on 'know that' knowledge. Further, it is stated that nurses in advanced roles are "knowledge brokers" because part of their work is to locate, evaluate, synthesize, and communicate knowledge to other clinical nurses on the team. As part of their position as knowledge brokers, advanced practice nurses may develop, apply, and evaluate nursing mid-range and practice theories, so contributing to the expansion of the nursing knowledge base for nursing practice.

REVIEW QUESTIONS

1. What are the primary roles of a nurse?
2. Explain some implications of the new nursing roles.
3. What is role theory?
4. Discuss the biomedical model on nursing roles.
5. What are the limitations of 'grand' theories?

MULTIPLE CHOICE QUESTIONS

1. Primary care is:

a. Care provided by GPs only.
b. The first point of contact for people seeking health care.
c. Care provided in hospices.
d. Care provided in the acute setting.

2. NHS Direct:

a Offers a 24-hour service over the telephone.
b. Offers a 24-hour service via the internet.
c. Offers a 24-hour service by GPs.
d. Offers advice to paramedics and accident and emergency staff.

3. Team nursing:

a. Has been phased out.
b. Lacks an evidence base.
c. Is practiced by teams of variously educated healthcare workers.
d. Is a substandard approach to care delivery?

4. A nurse's role is

a. To communicate with patients
b. To provide treatments, including medication
c. To support an individual emotionally
d. All of the above

5. Key nursing skills

a. Emotionally support
b. Show compassion and empathy
c. Ability to adapt to situations
d. All of the above

Answers to Multiple Choice Questions

1. (b) 2. (a) 3. (c) 4. (d) 5. (d)

REFERENCES

1. Acob, PhD, Joel Rey Ugsang, and WiwinMartiningsih. "Role Development Of Nurse Managers In The Changing Health Care Practice." JurnalNersdanKebidanan (Journal of Ners and Midwifery) 5, no. 1 (April 2018): 066–68.
2. Alleyne, Jergen, Ann Bonner, and Patricia B. Strasser. "Occupational Health Nurses' Roles, Credentials, and Continuing Education in Ontario, Canada." AAOHN Journal 57, no. 9 (September 2009): 389–95.
3. Armstrong-Stassen, Marjorie, Michelle Freeman, Sheila Cameron, and Dale Rajacic. "Nurse managers' role in older nurses' intention to stay." Journal of Health Organization and Management 29, no. 1 (March 2015): 55–74.
4. Harper-Femson, Lee Anne. "Nurse practitioners' role satisfaction." Electronic thesis or diss., National Library of Canada = Bibliothèquenationale du Canada, 1998. http://www.collectionscanada.ca/obj/s4/f2/dsk2/tape17/PQDD_0012/NQ35403.pdf.
5. Jacob, Elisabeth R., Lisa McKenna, and Angelo D'Amore. "Senior nurse role expectations of graduate registered and enrolled nurses on commencement to practice." Australian Health Review 38, no. 4 (2014): 432.
6. L., Evelyn, and Gonzales. "Burn Clinical Nurse Specialist/Nurse Clinician Roles and Role Development." Journal of Burn Care & Rehabilitation 8, no. 1 (January 1987): 25–27.
7. Osborne, Yvonne Therese, and res cand@acuedu au. "An Exploration of How Nurses Construct their Leadership Role During the Provision of Health Care." Australian Catholic University. School of Educational Leadership, 2006.
8. Roziers, Reinette. "Newly qualified nurses lived experience of role transition from student nurse to community service nurse a phenomenological study ReinetteRoziers." Master Thesis, University of Cape Town, 2012. http://hdl.handle.net/11427/2962.
9. Tsung, Pui-kee Peggy. "Nurses' role in smoking cessation knowledge, attitudes and behaviours /." Hong Kong : University of Hong Kong, 2002. http://sunzi.lib.hku.hk/hkuto/record.jsp?B26294825.
10. Widyasrini, JatiUjiSekti, and Sri Lestari. "Dual Role Conflict, Coping Stress, And Social Support As Nurses' Well-Being Predictor." JurnalPsikologi 19, no. 2 (June 2020): 174–87.

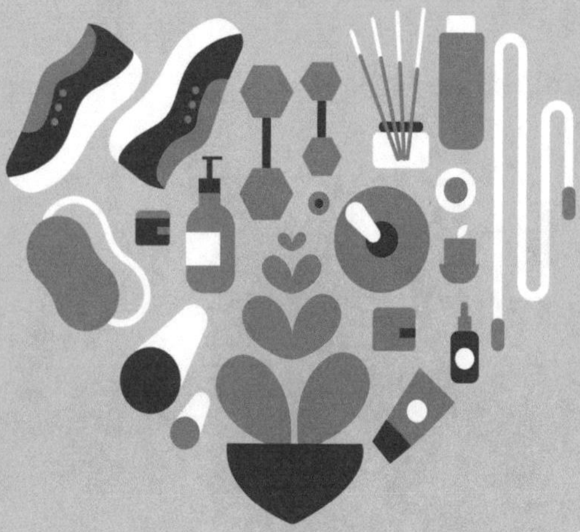

CHAPTER 4

HEALTH AND WELLNESS

"Wellness encompasses a healthy body, a sound mind, and a tranquil spirit. Enjoy the journey as you strive for wellness."

—Laurette Gagnon Beaulieu

INTRODUCTION

The primary objectives of the nurse as the caregiver are to promote health, to prevent illness, to restore health, and to facilitate coping with illness, disability, or death. These objectives aim to maximize the health of patients of all ages, in all environments, and in both health and disease. Health is more than the absence of disease; it is the dynamic process by which a person reaches his or her full potential. Additionally, it has varied meanings for many individuals. To provide holistic care, care that addresses the multiple dimensions that make up the full individual, the nurse must understand and respect each individual's concept of health and responses to sickness, as well as be knowledgeable about models of health and illness. Because of the current emphasis on health promotion and advocacy, the ongoing trend toward care being offered in the home and community, the rising number of older persons, and the increasing prevalence of chronic illnesses, the nurse's knowledge of health and illness is more vital than ever.

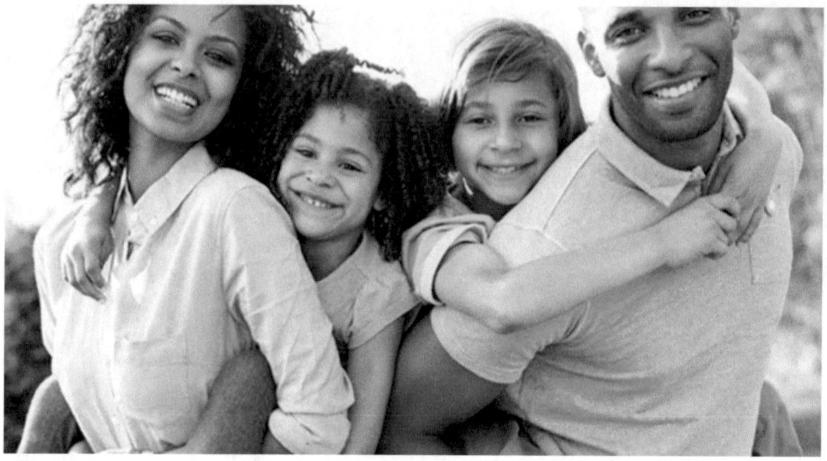

Learning Objectives

After completing the chapter, you will be able to accomplish the following:

- Describe the concepts of health, wellness
- Explain the concepts of illness and disease
- Define the factors affecting health and illness
- Summarize the health promotion and illness prevention
- Explain the models of health promotion and illness prevention
- Elaborate the nursing care to promote health and prevent illness

Key Terms

- Chronic illness
- Acute illness
- Physical care
- Emotional support
- Epidemic
- Medical care
- Blood pressure
- Cholesterol
- Skin cancer
- Health promotion model
- Health–illness continuum
- Holistic health

CONCEPTS OF HEALTH AND WELLNESS

A classic definition of health is that health is a state of complete physical, mental, and social well-being, not merely the absence of disease or illness. The health of the public is measured more globally by morbidity, how frequently a disease occurs and mortality, numbers of deaths. On a personal level, however, most individuals define health according to how they feel ("I feel really sick"), the absence or presence of symptoms of illness ("I have a terrible pain in my stomach"), or their ability to carry out activities of daily living ("I felt so much better that I got up and cooked supper").

Each person defines health in terms of his or her own values and beliefs. The family, culture, community, and society in which one lives also influence one's personal perception of health.

As defined by each individual, health is the integration of all human qualities, including the physical, mental, emotional, social, spiritual, and environmental aspects of the whole person. The nurse providing holistic nursing care must consider all these interdependent and interrelated aspects of the whole person (Fig. 4.1). Wellness, a concept frequently used synonymously with health, is the active pursuit of physical, mental, and emotional health through a lifestyle that encourages such. Model of high-level wellness as performing at one's maximum potential while maintaining environmental equilibrium and a sense of purpose. Dunn distinguished "wellness" from "good health," believing that good health is a passive condition in which the individual is not ill. Wellness is a state of increased activity, regardless of a person's

KEYWORD

Emotional health is about how we think and feel. It is about our sense of wellbeing, our ability to cope with life events and how we acknowledge our own emotions as well as those of others.

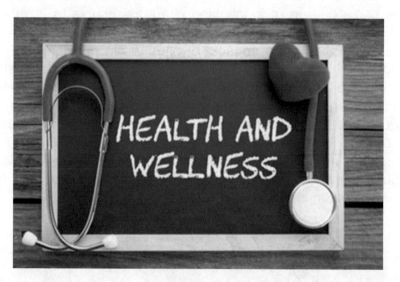

health. It also identified procedures that assist an individual understand who and what they are. Being (recognizing self as different and unique), belonging (being a part of a whole), becoming (growing and developing), and being fitting are the processes that comprise an individual's view of his or her own state of wellbeing (making personal choices to befit the self for the future). Dunn's approach urges the nurse to provide care for the whole person, taking into account all elements affecting the individual's state of being and striving for the individual's maximum potential.

Did you Know?

In the first decade of the 21st century, the conceptualization of health as an ability opened the door for self-assessments to become the main indicators to judge the performance of efforts aimed at improving human health.

CONCEPTS OF ILLNESS AND DISEASE

Disease is a medical term, meaning that there is a pathologic change in the structure or function of the body or mind. A disease is the cause of a person's illness; it is an aberrant process in which the person's degree of functioning changes relative to a previous level. This response is individual and impacted by self-perceptions, others' perceptions, the impacts of changes in physical form and function, the effects of those changes on roles and relationships, as well as cultural and spiritual values and beliefs. Traditionally, a physician diagnoses and treats a condition (although nurses with higher education increasingly do so), whereas nurses focus on the patient. However, the terms are frequently interchanged. It is essential for nurses to keep in mind that despite having a disease or injury, a patient may attain optimal functioning and quality of life and consider themselves healthy.

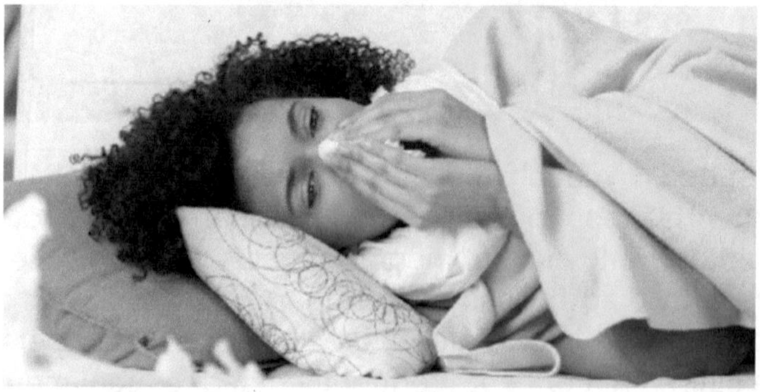

Classifications of Illness

Illnesses are classified as either acute or chronic. A person may have an acute illness, a chronic illness, or both at the same time; for example, an adult with diabetes (a chronic illness) may also have appendicitis (an acute illness).

Acute Illness and Illness Behaviors

Acute illness is characterized by a rapid onset of symptoms and a brief duration. Simple acute illnesses, such as the common cold or diarrhea, typically do not require medical treatment because they may be treated with self-medication and over-the-counter drugs.

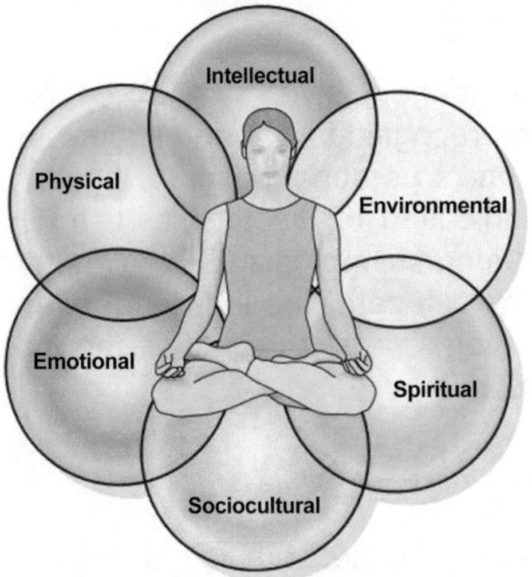

Figure 4.1. The human dimensions. All of these interdependent parts compose the whole person.

If medical care is required, a specific treatment with medications (e.g., antibiotics for pneumonia) or surgical procedures (e.g., an appendectomy for appendicitis) usually return the person to normal functioning.

When a person develops an acute disease, various symptoms may manifest in stages. These behaviors are how individuals cope with the function-altering effects of the disease. They are unique to the individual and are impacted by age, gender, family values, economic situation, culture, degree of education, and mental health.

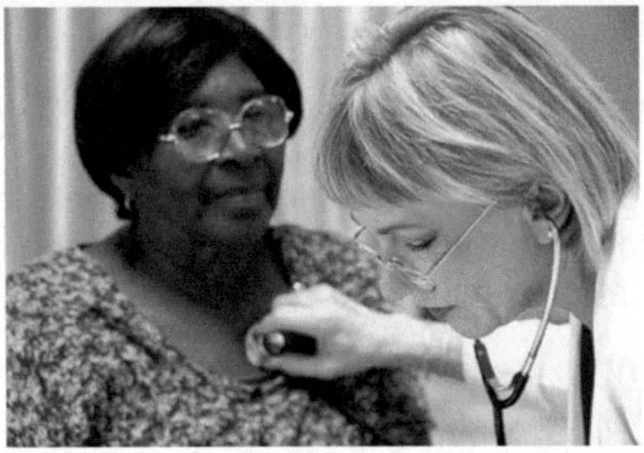

Figure 4.2. The nurse is assessing the patient as a basis for teaching healthy heart behaviors.

There is no set timeline for the onset of stages-of-illness behaviors, which might emerge quickly or gradually. Throughout all stages, nursing functions remain consistent. In all phases, the nurse acknowledges the patient as an individual, provides nursing care based on the patient's priority requirements, and encourages recovery by providing physical care, emotional support, and health education (Fig. 4.2).

Stage 1: Experiencing Symptoms

KEYWORD

Emotional support is showing care and compassion for another person. It may include actions such as helping a person call a therapist or giving a hug to a crying friend.

How do people define themselves as "sick"? Typically, the first sign of a disease is the recognition of one or more symptoms that are inconsistent with one's personal notion of health. Although pain is the most major indication of disease, a rash, fever, bleeding, or cough are also common symptoms. If the symptoms are temporary or are alleviated by self-care, the individual often takes no further action. If the symptoms persist, however, the individual advances to the next stage.

Stage 2: Assuming the Sick Role

The individual now describes oneself or herself as sick, seeks external confirmation of this experience, abandons usual activities, and assumes a "sick role." The majority of patients at this stage concentrate on their symptoms and body functioning. Depending on individual health beliefs and practices, the individual may opt to do nothing, purchase over-the-counter drugs to alleviate symptoms, or seek medical evaluation and treatment. When a healthcare provider diagnoses and prescribes therapy for a disease, it is recognized as legitimate in our culture. When assistance from a healthcare provider is sought, the individual becomes a patient and advances to the subsequent phase.

Stage 3: Assuming a Dependent Role

This phase is defined by the patient's acceptance of the diagnosis and adherence to the specified treatment plan. The individual conforms to the opinions of others, frequently needs assistance with daily activities, and demands emotional support through acceptance, approval, physical proximity, and protection.

If the ailment is severe (such as a heart attack or stroke), the patient may seek care in a hospital. If the symptoms can be managed by the patient or family on their own or with the help of home care providers, the patient is cared for at home. To encourage adherence to the treatment plan, the patient must have effective connections with caregivers, illness awareness, and a tailored care plan. The patient's responses to care rely on a number of variables, including the severity of the sickness, the patient's level of fear of the disease, the loss of roles, the support of others, and previous experiences with illness care. Both caregivers and family members anticipate the patient to recover and resume routine responsibilities.

KEYWORD

Rehabilitation is set of interventions designed to optimize functioning and reduce disability in individuals with health conditions in interaction with their environment.

Stage 4: Achieving Recovery and Rehabilitation

Recovery and rehabilitation may begin in the hospital and end at home, or may be completed entirely at a rehabilitation facility or at home. The majority of patients complete this final behavior stage at home. During this phase, the individual relinquishes the role of dependent and resumes normal activities and duties. If health education is included in the plan of care, the individual may return to health at a higher level of functioning and health than before the illness.

Chronic Illness

Chronic illness is a broad term that encompasses many different physical and mental alterations in health, with one or more of the following characteristics:

- It is a permanent change.
- It causes, or is caused by, irreversible alterations in normal anatomy and physiology.
- It requires special patient education for rehabilitation.
- It requires a long period of care or support.

Many chronic illnesses have phases of remission (when the disease is present, but the individual does not feel symptoms) and exacerbation (when symptoms worsen orthe symptoms of the disease reappear). Examples of common chronic diseases include cardiovascular disease, diabetes, lung ailments, and arthritis.

The annual cost of chronic illness in the United States is estimated to exceed $1 trillion. Chronic diseases are the biggest cause of death worldwide. In light of this, the health promotion and disease prevention efforts outlined later in this chapter are even more crucial to nursing care. Rising numbers of older persons, lifestyle choices (such as smoking and drug use), environmental factors (increasing air and water pollution), and the AIDS epidemic are current trends that contribute to an increase in chronic diseases. In the future, more individuals with chronic illnesses will require nursing care. Although not all people with a chronic illness require care, all chronically sick individuals must accept certain conditions of life in order to manage their illness on a daily basis for the remainder of their lives. People with a chronic illness frequently experience loss or change in bodily structure or function, worry about finances, status, roles, and dignity, and must confront the potential of an earlier death. Seven of the top 10 main causes of death in the United States are chronic illnesses. (heart disease, cancer, stroke, respiratory disease, diabetes, Alzheimer's disease, and kidney disease)

KEYWORD

Chronic illness refers to a long-term medical condition that persists for an extended period, typically longer than three months.

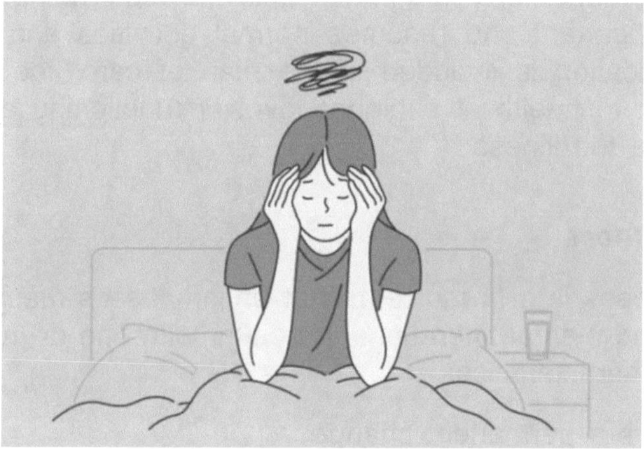

To successfully adapt to a chronic illness, a person must learn to live as normally as possible and keep a positive self-concept and feeling of hope, despite symptoms and treatments that may make them feel different from others. Frequently, modifications must be made to a person's activities of daily living, relationships, and self-care routines, and it is essential that he or she maintains a sense of control over his or her life and recommended therapies.

Nurses offer care for chronically sick patients of all ages in a variety of settings, including homes, hospitals, clinics, long-term care facilities, and institutions. Regardless of the age of the patient, the impacts and demands of the illness, or the setting, the nurse must make every effort to improve the health of patients with chronic illness, with an emphasis on what is still feasible rather than what is no longer possible.

Effects of Illness on the Family

The majority of nursing care is provided to patients with a support system, typically family members. When an illness arises, both the patient's and the family's duties alter. For instance, a chronic illness may necessitate lifelong modifications to the patient's function or lifestyle, repeated hospitalizations, economic difficulties, and limited social connections within the family. Likewise, the responses of family members to a disease are unique. Some family members desire constant contact with the sick, while others may avoid visiting. Parents of a sick kid frequently respond with resentment, overprotection, and extreme worry, and family members of patients requiring intensive care frequently experience feelings of isolation and fear. In both instances, they may experience remorse and imagine the worst-case scenario.

KEYWORD

Holistic care refers to the provision of care to patients that are based on a mutual understanding of their physical, psychological, emotional, and spiritual dimensions.

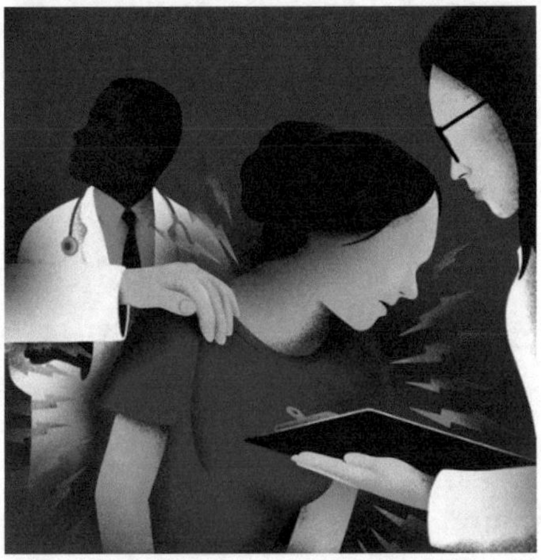

FACTORS AFFECTING HEALTH AND ILLNESS

Many factors influence a person's health status, health beliefs, and health practices. These elements may be internal or external to the individual, and the individual may or may not have conscious influence over them. To plan and administer holistic care, the nurse must comprehend how these variables affect the behavior of both healthy and ill patients.

Basic Human Needs

A basic human need is a necessity for the emotional and physiological well and survival of humans. A person whose requirements are met may be deemed healthy, whereas a person with one or more unmet needs is at a greater risk of becoming unwell.

The Human Dimensions

Remember

Treating only the body will not necessarily restore optimal health. In addition to physical needs, nurses must also consider clients' psychological, sociocultural, developmental, and spiritual needs.

The elements that influence a person's health–illness status, health beliefs, and health behaviors–have to do with the individual's human dimensions (refer back to Fig. 4.1). Each dimension interacts with the others and determines the health and illness behaviors of the individual. The nursing assessments of the patient's strengths and weaknesses in each domain are utilized to construct a personalized and comprehensive plan of care.

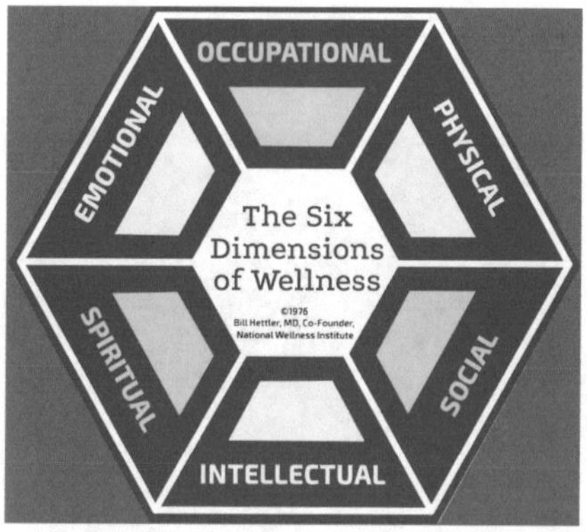

Physical Dimension

The physical dimension consists of genetic inheritance, age, stage of development, race, and gender. These factors have a significant impact on the individual's health state and health practices. As examples, inherited genetic disorders include Down syndrome, hemophilia, cystic fibrosis, and color blindness. The toddler is at a greater risk for drowning, and the adolescent and young adult male are at a greater risk for automobile crashes due to excessive speed. There are specific racial traits for disease, such as sickle cell anemia, hypertension, and stroke; and a young woman who has a mother and a grandmother with breast cancer is more likely to have an annual clinical breast examination and mammogram.

Emotional Dimension

The manner in which the mind impacts bodily function and reacts to bodily conditions also affects health. Long-term stress impacts physiological systems, and anxiety influences health behaviors;

on the other hand, calm acceptance and relaxation can alter the body's responses to illness. A student who constantly gets diarrhea before exams and an adolescent who begins experimenting with drugs are instances of the negative effects of emotions. Among the good impacts of emotions are the reduction of surgical pain through relaxation techniques and the reduction of blood pressure through biofeedback abilities.

KEYWORD

Health education is any combination of learning experiences designed to facilitate voluntary actions conducive to health.

Intellectual Dimension

The intellectual dimension includes cognitive aptitude, educational history, and past experiences. These factors affect responses to health education and reactions to nursing care during illness. They also have a significant impact on health-related behaviors. Instances involving this dimension include a young college student with diabetes who adheres to a diabetic diet but continues to drink beer and eat pizza with friends several times per week, and a middle-aged man who stops taking his hypertension medication after experiencing unpleasant side effects.

Environmental Dimension

The environment has numerous effects on health and disease. Aspects of the environmental dimension include housing, sanitation, climate, and contamination of air, food, and water. The deaths of older persons due to inadequate heating and cooling, the increased incidence of asthma and respiratory difficulties in large cities with smog, and the increased incidence of skin cancer in hot, sunny regions of the world are examples of environmental causes of sickness.

Sociocultural Dimension

The health practices and beliefs of an individual are heavily influenced by their socioeconomic status, lifestyle, family, and culture. Low-income groups are less likely to seek preventative medical treatment, but high-income groups are more susceptible to stress-related behaviors and sickness. The family and culture to which a person belongs influence his or her patterns of life and beliefs on health and illness; such patterns are frequently unchangeable. Personal hygiene, dietary habits, lifestyle choices, and mental stability are all affected by these variables. Other sociocultural situations that influence health and illness include an adolescent who sees nothing wrong with smoking or drinking because her parents do the same, parents of a sick infant who do not seek medical care because they lack health insurance, a single parent (who was abused as a child) who physically abuses her own young son, and an individual of Asian descent who uses herbal remedies and acupuncture to treat an illness.

Spiritual Dimension

Spiritual ideas and values are crucial components of an individual's health and sickness behaviors. It is essential that nurses respect these values and recognize their significance for each patient. Examples of spiritual influences on healthcare include the Roman Catholic requirement of baptism for both live births and stillborn babies, Kosher dietary laws prohibiting the consumption of pork and shellfish, practiced by Orthodox and Conservative Jews, and Jehovah's Witnesses' opposition to blood transfusion.

TIPS

The effects of illness on a person's roles, independence, and relationships with significant individuals might alter their sense of self.

Self-Concept

A person's self-concept, which includes both how he or she thinks about him or herself (self-esteem) and how he or she perceives his or her physical self, also influences health and illness (body image). Self-concept comprises both physical and emotional components and is a significant determinant in how an individual responds to stress and sickness, engages in self-care, and interacts with others. Past experiences, interpersonal interactions, physical and cultural factors, and education all contribute to the formation of an individual's self-concept. It contains an individual's judgments of their own strengths and limitations.

Risk Factors for Illness or Injury

A risk factor is something that raises the likelihood of a person becoming unwell or injured. As with other aspects of health and disease, risk factors are frequently interconnected. Risk factors can be further classified as modifiable (changeable, such quitting smoking) or nonmodifiable (unable to be changed, such as a family history of cancer). As the number of risk factors rises, so does the likelihood of becoming unwell. For instance, an obese CEO who is under pressure to enhance sales smokes and consumes excessive amounts of alcohol. These variables, coupled with a family history of heart disease, increase this person's likelihood of developing a condition.

Table 4.1 below outlines the six primary types of risk variables.

Table 4.1: Major Areas of Risk Factors

Risk Factor	Examples
Age	School-aged children are at high risk for communicable diseases. After menopause, women are more likely to develop cardiovascular disease.
Genetic factors	A family history of cancer or diabetes predisposes a person to developing the disease.
Physiologic factors	Obesity increases the possibility of heart disease. Pregnancy places increased risk on both the mother and the developing fetus.
Health habits	Smoking increases the probability of lung cancer. Poor nutrition can lead to a variety of health problems.
Lifestyle	Multiple sexual relationships increase the risk for sexually transmitted infections (e.g., gonorrhea or acquired immunodeficiency syndrome). Events that increase stress (e.g., divorce, retirement, work-related pressure) may precipitate accidents or illness.
Environment	Working and living environments (such as hazardous materials and poor sanitation) may contribute to disease.

HEALTH PROMOTION AND ILLNESS PREVENTION

Health promotion is an individual's conduct that is driven by the desire to improve health and health potential. In contrast, illness/disease prevention is conduct that is driven by a desire to avoid or detect disease, or to sustain functioning within the limitations of illness or disability. Tradition describes health promotion and disease prevention initiatives as occurring at the primary, secondary, and tertiary levels. The definitions and examples of nursing actions for each level are presented in Table 4.2 below.

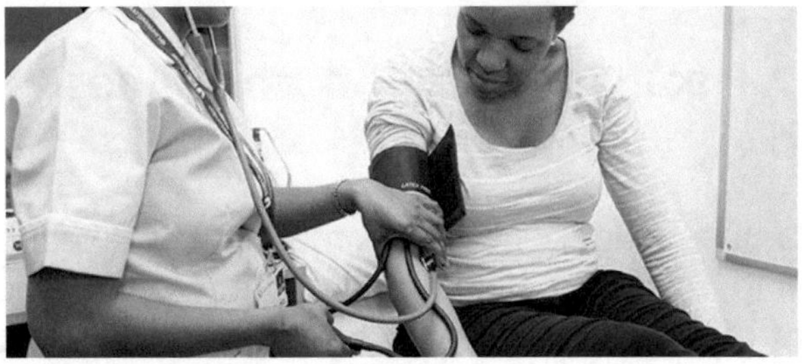

Primary Health Promotion and Illness Prevention

The purpose of primary health promotion and illness prevention is to promote health and prevent the onset of disease or harm. Primary-level nursing activities may focus on people or groups. Primary-level initiatives include vaccination clinics, family planning services, poison control information dissemination, and accident-prevention education. Other nurse treatments include education about a healthy diet, the significance of regular exercise, industrial and agricultural safety, the use of seatbelts, and safer sexual practices.

Assessments of health risks are an integral aspect of primary health promotion and preventive care. A health-risk assessment is an evaluation of the entire individual. The resulting "picture" of the individual identifies areas at risk for sickness or injury as well as places that promote health. There are numerous evaluation methods, but they all take a holistic approach to health, focusing on lifestyle and behaviors. As you work with patients to provide care, use this self-assessment to assist them in evaluating their current state of health and potential health concerns, as well as in adopting a healthier lifestyle through the recommended lifestyle habits that promote health.

Remember

Nurses' work has traditionally been influenced by Western medical models of health that focus on the organic nature and cause of mental and physical disease rather than the influence of internal and external variables on the health of the whole person.

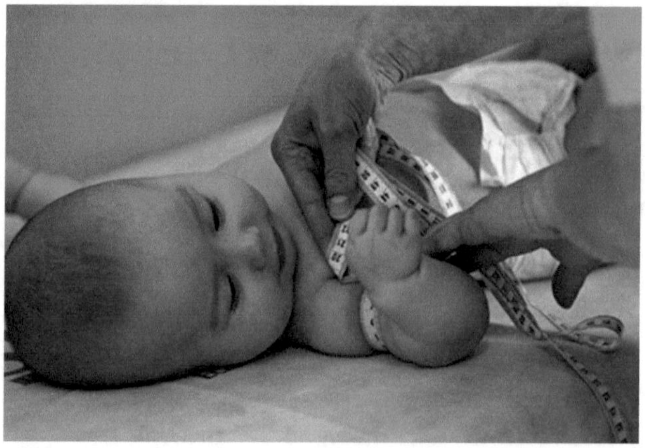

Secondary Health Promotion and Illness Prevention

The emphasis of secondary health promotion and disease prevention is on screening for early disease detection and rapid diagnosis and treatment of individuals who are diagnosed. The objectives of secondary preventive care are to recognize a disease, reverse or lessen the severity of the disease, or provide a cure, and to return the individual as rapidly as possible to optimal health. Assessing children for proper growth and development and encouraging frequent medical, dental, and eye examinations are examples of nursing duties at this level. Other activities include tests (e.g., for blood pressure, cholesterol, and skin cancer), advising gynecologic checkups and mammograms for women when age-appropriate, and educating men on how to perform testicular self-examination. At the secondary level, direct nursing care interventions include providing prescriptions and caring for wounds.

Table 4.2: Examples of nursing activities by level of health promotion and preventive care

Level	Topic
Primary	Weight loss Diet Exercise Smoking cessation Alcohol consumption Drugs Farm safety Seat belts and child safety seats Immunizations Water treatment Safer sex practices Parenting
Secondary	Screenings (Blood pressure, cholesterol, glaucoma, HIV, skin cancer) Pap smears Mammograms Testicular examinations Family counseling

Tertiary	Medications Medical therapy Surgical treatment Rehabilitation Physical therapy Occupational therapy Job training

Tertiary Health Promotion and Illness Prevention

KEYWORD

Physical therapy is commonly used in rehabilitation settings, such as post-surgical or post-injury recovery, to restore function, reduce pain, and improve mobility.

After a disease has been detected and treated, tertiary health promotion and disease prevention are implemented to lessen disability and assist patients in regaining their full level of function. Teaching a patient with diabetes how to recognize and prevent complications, using physical therapy to prevent contractures in patients who have suffered a stroke or spinal cord injury, and referring a woman to a support group after breast removal due to cancer are examples of tertiary-level nursing activities. Monitoring the patient's reaction to prescribed therapy and providing patients with services to assist recovery or improve quality of life while living with the symptoms of an illness or accident are essential functions of nurses.

MODELS OF HEALTH PROMOTION AND ILLNESS PREVENTION

Models of why and how individuals engage in health-promoting and disease-preventalive activities are valuable in assisting healthcare professionals to comprehend health-related behaviors and adjust care to varied economic and cultural backgrounds. This knowledge can be used to overcome barriers to health caused by disparities in care caused by factors such as the increasing number of people without health insurance, a predicted increase in minority populations, and a lack of accessible and essential healthcare services for low-income and rural populations.

The Health Belief Model

Most localities offer free or low-cost screenings and health education materials to aid in the early diagnosis of disease and promote healthy living. Why then don't more individuals utilize these services or alter their lifestyles? The prevalent health belief model, which explains health behaviors, can be utilized to answer this question.

The health belief model is concerned with what individuals perceive or think to be true regarding their health. This model is based on three aspects of individual perceptions of illness threat: perceived susceptibility to a disease, perceived severity of a disease, and perceived benefits of action.

KEYWORD

Health belief model is a social psychological health behavior change model developed to explain and predict health-related behaviors, particularly in regard to the uptake of health services.

Perceived susceptibility to a disease is the idea that an individual will get an illness or will not. It ranges from a fear of developing a disease to an outright denial that certain habits can cause illness. For instance, one cigarette smoker may believe he or she is at risk for lung cancer and quit, whereas another smoker may believe smoking poses no severe risk and continue to smoke.

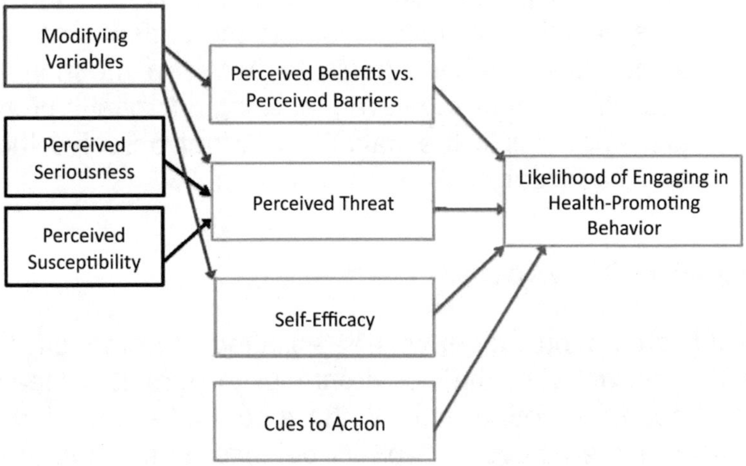

Perceived seriousness of a condition refers to the threat to health caused by the disease and its impact on the lifestyle of the individual. This component relates to the individual's knowledge of the disease and can lead to a change in health behavior. A smoker is more likely to quit if he or she feels that lung cancer can result in physical incapacity or death, so affecting his or her ability to work and care for the family.

Perceived advantages of action refers to how effective a person believes steps will be in preventing disease. This element is influenced by the individual's conviction that a prescribed activity will prevent or modify the disease, as well as the individual's assessment of the behavior's cost and negative consequences (compared with not taking any action). For instance, a person may believe that quitting smoking will avoid future respiratory issues and that initial withdrawal symptoms are surmountable; as a result, the individual may quit smoking.

Demographic variables (such as age and gender), sociopsychological variables (such as personality and peer group pressure), and structural variables can influence an individual's health beliefs (such as knowledge and prior contact with the disease). These factors determine the perceived advantages of preventative activity minus the perceived disadvantages of preventive action. Cues to action are also modifying factors and include actions such as the advice of others, mass-media campaigns, literature, appointment-reminder phone calls or postcards, and a significant other's illness. Individual views and moderating factors contribute to the chance of implementing a recommended preventive health measure.

KEYWORD

Health promotion model notes that each person has unique personal characteristics and experiences that affect subsequent actions.

When educating people about health and illness, the health belief model is effective. You can evaluate the patient's associated beliefs and mutually establish goals to assist in meeting health needs in a realistic manner. However, teaching and health promotion initiatives are worthless if the patient does not perceive them as important and necessary.

The Health Promotion Model

The health promotion model was established to demonstrate how individuals interact with their environment in pursuit of health. To motivate health-promoting activity, the model integrates individual features and experiences as well as behavior-specific information and beliefs. The model's components can be utilized to create and implement nursing interventions that promote the health of individuals, families, and communities.

Individual qualities and experiences can be utilized to predict whether or not a person would adopt and utilize health-related habits. If a behavior is repeated and becomes habitual, it is more likely to occur again. Personal biological, psychological, and social characteristics, such as age, gender, strength, self-esteem, perceived health status, concept of health, acculturation, and socioeconomic level, are all predictive of a particular health-related behavior. A person with strong self-esteem, a healthy self-perception, and a sufficient income may be less likely to use alcohol or tobacco and more likely to consume a balanced diet and engage in regular exercise. In contrast, a person with low self-esteem, a fatalistic outlook on health, and a limited socioeconomic foundation may be more prone to have bad nutrition, never exercise, and use addictive substances.

Considered to be important motivators for engaging in health-promoting actions include behavior-specific knowledge, attitudes, and relationships. These include the idea that a given health behavior will have a beneficial consequence, the belief that one has the ability and competence to engage in health behaviors, and the belief that one is influenced by the interpersonal impacts of others (especially family, peers, and healthcare providers). Situational variables, such as smoking bans, also affect health-related behaviors. Typically, barriers to action, such as beliefs of unavailability, annoyance, expense, or difficulty, result in behavior avoidance. Initiating a health-related behavior begins with committing to a plan of action, followed by the development of methods to execute the desired behavior. Inability to maintain the behavior may be the result of competing demands. A person may, for instance, adopt a low-fat diet yet "give in" to the convenience of fast food. The result of the model is health-related behavior aimed at achieving favorable health outcomes and experiences throughout the lifespan.

KEYWORD

Health–illness continuum describes how wellbeing is more than simply an absence of illness , but also incorporates the individuals mental and emotional health.

The Health–Illness Continuum

The health–illness continuum is one method for measuring an individual's state of health. This paradigm considers health as a state that is continually changing, with optimal health and mortality

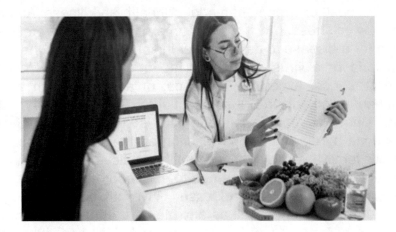

being at opposite ends of a continuum (Figure 4.3). This continuum depicts the ever-changing state of health as an individual adapts to changes in their internal and external environments in order to maintain a level of health. A patient with cancer, for instance, may perceive themselves at different positions on the continuum at any one time, depending on how well the patient believes he or she is coping with the illness.

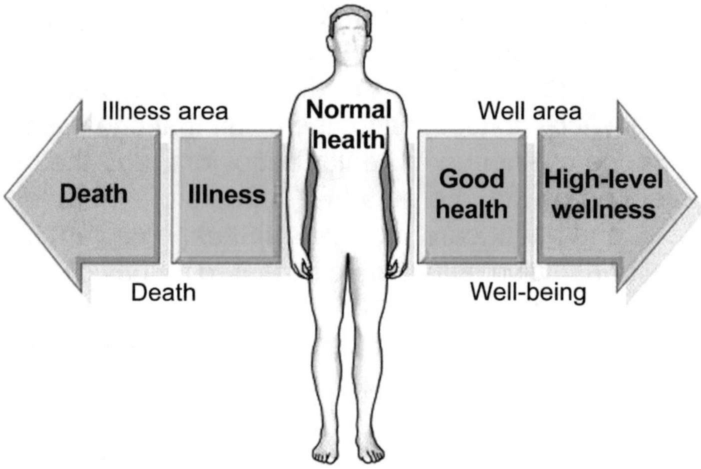

Figure 4.3: The health–illness continuum.

The Agent–Host–Environment Model

Examining the origins of disease in an individual is facilitated by the agent–host–environment model of health and illness. An agent is a factor or stressor in the environment that must be present or missing for a disease to develop. For instance, the component may be bacteria or a virus, a chemical agent, or a form of radiation whose presence, excessive presence, or absence (such as in a vitamin-deficiency disorder) is essential for the development of an illness. A host is a biological entity that is susceptible to infection or influence by an agent. The reaction of the host is impacted by the host's family history, age, and health practices. The environment comprises all elements external to the body that increase or decrease the likelihood of disease. Physical, social, biological, and cultural aspects, as well as any others that affect health, may be included. A person with poor dietary habits and little sleep, for instance, is more susceptible to infection during an influenza outbreak. If the individual is also immunocompromised (as in AIDS), the risk is significantly higher. Figure 4.4 depicts how each of the agent–host–environment factors influences and is influenced by the others. Constant interaction between these elements may increase the chance of sickness. When the factors are in equilibrium, health is preserved; when they are out of equilibrium, sickness develops. Consequently, health is a dynamic state.

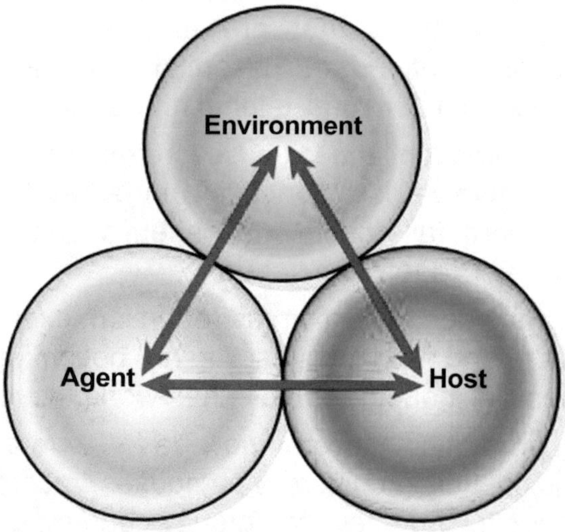

Figure 4.4. The agent–host–environment triangle.

NURSING CARE TO PROMOTE HEALTH AND PREVENT ILLNESS

The current focus on health promotion and illness prevention at local, state, national, and global levels is important to nursing.

Nurses must maintain their personal health in order to provide good nursing care to others. Good personal health allows nurses to not only practice more effectively, but also serve as role models for patients and their families. Nurses can assist patients in adopting new health behaviors by demonstrating those practices themselves. When their personal needs are not satisfied, it is difficult for nurses to be sensitive to the needs of patients. Due to the fact that no one is always in perfect health, it is crucial that nurses preparing for professional practice spend time getting to know themselves. From this self-knowledge should come a commitment to actively pursue holistic health.

As the 21st century progresses, resources for healthcare practices for self and others and retaining awareness of healthcare trends can assist in improving health and advocating for patients and families of all ages and in all situations.

- Telehealth practice, in which electronically transmitted clinical consultation and treatment has increased access to care for persons living in rural or underserved areas of the country, is utilized for health promotion and disease preventive efforts. It is assisting in reducing the number of hospitalizations that are needless. The American Nurses Association was essential in obtaining Medicare reimbursement for rural telehealth services.
- Health promotion and disease prevention education and activities involve risk reduction and behavior modification; activities are tailored to the patient's unique health risk environment, age, and gender.
- Programs emphasizing stress reduction, exercise, smoking cessation, and weight counseling are becoming increasingly prevalent in industries and other workplaces.
- Health promotion sites can now be found in a vast array of settings, including university campuses, retirement centers, day schools, churches, community centers, grocery stores, and sites for senior nutrition.
- Healthcare services must be provided in nontraditional settings to provide screening and education to homeless, migrant, and carnival workers, among others.

KEYWORD

Medicare reimbursement is the process by which a doctor or health facility receives funds for providing medical services to a Medicare beneficiary.

REVIEW QUESTIONS

1. What do you observe about the effects of the illness in relation to the patient's age, type of illness (e.g., AIDS versus cancer), gender, and family role?
2. What are the concepts of illness and disease?
3. Define the acute illness and illness behaviors.
4. How many factors affect health and illness?
5. Describe the models of health promotion and illness prevention.

MULTIPLE CHOICE QUESTIONS

1. Of the following statements, which is most true of health and illness?

a. Health and illness are the same for all people.
b. Health and illness are individually defined by each person.
c. People with acute illnesses are actually healthy.
d. People with chronic illnesses have poor health beliefs.

2. A nurse has volunteered to give influenza injections at a local clinic. What level of care is he demonstrating?

a. Tertiary
b. Secondary
c. Primary
d. Promotive

3. A nurse's neighbor tells her, "I have a high temperature, feel awful, and I am not going to work." What stage of illness behavior is the neighbor exhibiting?

a. Experiencing symptoms
b. Assuming the sick role
c. Assuming a dependent role
d. Achieving recovery and rehabilitation

4. A nurse is caring for a patient with heart failure, a chronic illness. Which of the following characteristics is not a part of chronic illness?

a. Permanent change in body structure or function
b. Self-treatment that relieves symptoms
c. Long period of treatment and care
d. Often has remissions and exacerbations

5. The agent–host–environment model of health and illness is based on what concept?

a. Risk factors

b. Infectious diseases

c. Behaviors to promote health

d. Stages of illness

Answers to Multiple Choice Questions

1. (b) 2. (c) 3. (b) 4. (b) 5. (a)

REFERENCES

1. Condon, M., & Welker-Hood, K. (2007). Environment, health, and safety. American Nurse Today, 2(6), 56.
2. Delgado, C. (2007). Sense of coherence, spirituality, stress, and quality of life in chronic illness. Journal of Nursing Scholarship, 39(3), 229–234.
3. Dunn, H. (1980). High-level wellness. Thorofare, NJ: Slack, Inc.
4. Edelman, C., &Mandle, C. (2006). Health promotion throughout the life span (5th ed.). St. Louis, MO: Mosby.
5. How to lower your health risks, at any age. (2008). Consumer Reports on Health, 20(8), 1, 45.
6. Leavell, H., & Clark, E. G. (1965). Preventive medicine for the doctor in the community (3rd ed.). New York: McGraw Hill.
7. Mason, D. (2005). The state of the science: Focus on chronic illness. American Journal of Nursing, 105(2), 27–28.
8. Murray, R. B., Zentner, J. P., &Yakimo, R. (2009). Health promotion strategies through the lifespan (8th ed.). Upper Saddle River, NJ: Pearson Prentice Hall.
9. National Center for Health Statistics. (2008). Deaths—leading causes. Available at http://www.cdc.gov/nchs/FASTATS/ lcod.htm
10. Pender, N., Murdaugh, C., & Parsons, M. (2006). Health promotion in nursing practice (6th ed.). Upper Saddle River, NJ: Pearson Prentice Hall.
11. Rosenstock, I. (1974). Historical origin of the health belief model. Health Education Monographs, 2, 334.
12. Sheer, B. (2007). Nursing and the impact of worldwide poverty. Topics in Advanced Practice Nursing eJournal, 7(3). Available at http://www.medscape.com/viewarticle/564102

13. Sobering statistics. (2008). American Journal of Nursing, 108(1), 22.
14. Stanhope, M., & Lancaster, J. (2006). Foundations of nursing in the community. (2nd ed.). St. Louis: Mosby.
15. Suchman, E. (1965). Stages of illness and medical care. Journal of Health and Human Behavior, 6, 114.
16. U.S. Department of Health and Human Services. (2000). Healthy people 2010. Washington, DC: Author.
17. World Health Organization. (1974). Constitution of the World Health Organization: Chronicle of the World Health Organization. Geneva: Author.

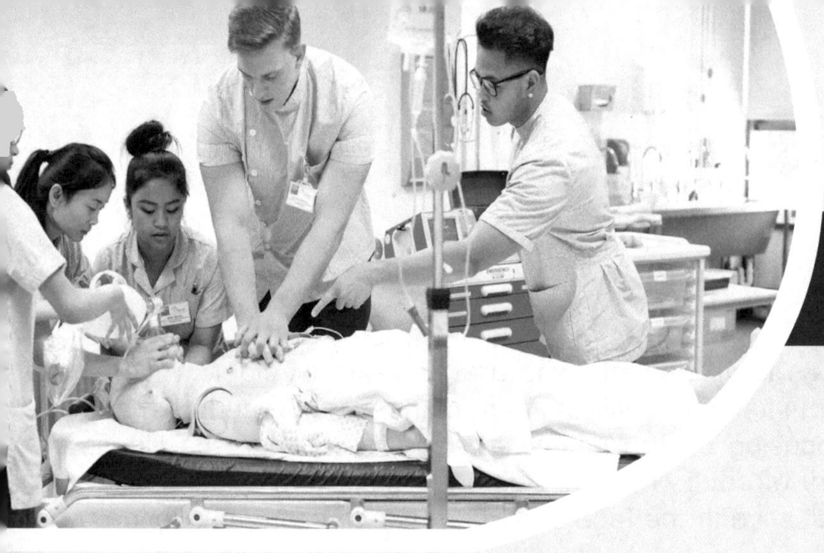

CHAPTER 5

ADULT NURSING

"Nurses dispense comfort, compassion, and caring without even a prescription."

—Val Saintsbury

INTRODUCTION

Adult nurses provide treatment for patients with a range of health issues, from minor accidents and disorders to acute and chronic illnesses and diseases. Utilizing care plans, care procedures, and assessments, and analyzing and focusing on the patient's needs rather than the illness or condition, they promote healing.

The patient care unit is the part of the hospital where the patient receives medical and nursing care and treatment, and where he or she resides during his or her hospitalization.

The environment must be kept safe, pleasant, clean, and organized for the patient's physical and mental wellness. Constant effort is required to attain and maintain the required degree of order and cleanliness.

We frequently visit the hospital when our friends or family members require medical care. Adult nursing personnel are directly involved in determining your health condition and giving therapy; they are the first thing we encounter. They provide care for patients with situations ranging from minor accidents and ailments to acute and chronic diseases and illnesses. If you are interested in nursing, you must first determine the area of nursing you wish to pursue. There are four branches of nursing:

- Adult nursing
- Pediatric nursing
- Mental health nursing
- Learning disability nursing

The primary focus of adult nurses is on patients who are 18 years or older, while all patients must be able to receive safe, vital care. Utilizing care plans, care procedures, and assessments, and analyzing and focusing on the patient's needs rather than the illness or condition, they aid in the recovery of adult patients. Being an adult nurse requires the ability to maintain composure and initiative in the face of numerous interesting challenges.

Learning Objectives

After completing the chapter, you will be able to accomplish the following:

- Define adult nursing
- Gain knowledge to become an adult nurse
- What to expect as an adult nurse
- Discuss the enrolment requirements to study adult nursing
- Explain the role of nursing in adult social care

Key-Terms

- Physician
- Covid-19 pandemic
- Physiotherapist
- Occupational therapist
- Pharmacist
- Radiographer
- Healthcare assistant
- Communication skill
- Daycare center
- Primary Care Networks

ADULT NURSING

Adult nursing students anticipate learning practical skills and processes. Adult nurses care for elderly and young adults with a variety of chronic and acute health issues. Depending on your experience and education, as a nurse in the adult branch you will be at the heart of a multidisciplinary team that includes physicians, physiotherapists, occupational therapists, pharmacists, radiographers, healthcare assistants, and others.

Special Demands

- Nursing students will need the presence of mind and flexibility to juggle the needs of a number of individuals at the same time.
- Communication skills are essential for nursing success. Students pursuing a degree in nursing must possess the interpersonal skills necessary to put patients at rest in stressful and often difficult situations.
- As a nursing student, you will also experience the immense gratification of knowing that your contribution to decreasing suffering and increasing the health of those in your care is truly meaningful.
- The adult branch of nursing is ideal for individuals who prefer to work in a busy, interdisciplinary team, but who are also capable of taking initiative when necessary.
- You must be highly alert and able to determine what is best for the patient because there is a great deal to learn in a challenging, rapidly changing workplace.
- The willingness to assume responsibility for the well-being of others is fundamental, as is the commitment to lifelong learning.

KEYWORD

Healthcare assistants make sure the patient experience is as comfortable and stress-free as possible.

BECOME AN ADULT NURSE

There are numerous reasons to pursue a career in adult nursing. First and foremost, becoming an adult nurse entails improving and saving the lives of others via expertise and diligence. You will have the opportunity to impact the life of a patient you have never met from day one. In addition, it encompasses many areas of healthcare, and you get to interact with individuals of varying ages and backgrounds, which can be quite stimulating.

If you're looking for a career in which you can put your passion to serve people to excellent use, have a broad career and more opportunities in the workplace, being an adult nurse is a great option. In addition, it is commonly stated that "you need a physician to diagnose you, but a nurse to save your life."

TIPS

Nurses usually work within a multidisciplinary team but are the main point of contact for patients, often providing the most consistent care.

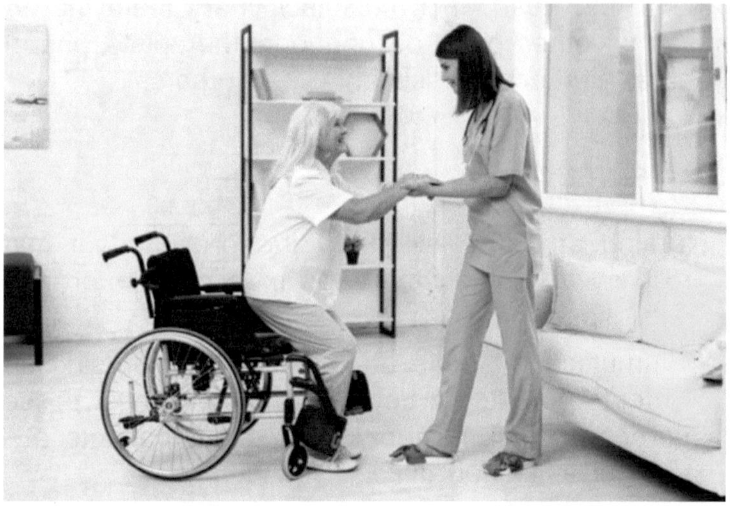

Career Overview of an Adult Nurse

Adult nursing is a dynamic field of work. These careers involve more than just caring for patients and their families. There are numerous responsibilities, such as handling paperwork, assisting physicians with patient diagnosis, and offering guidance and follow-up care, as well as numerous career options, profitable employment sectors, and salaries.

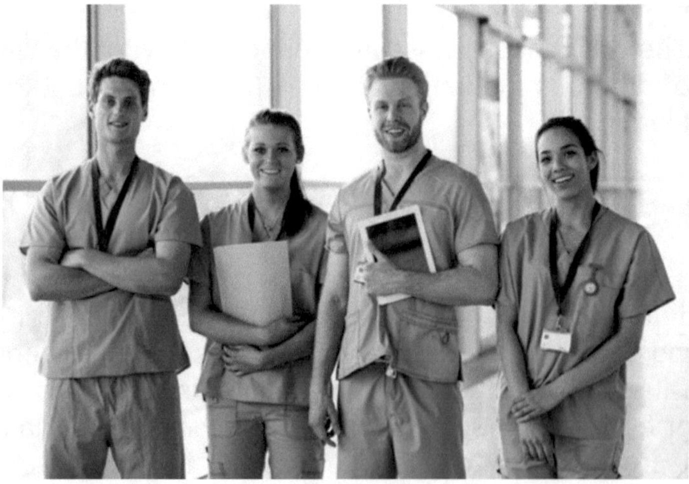

With Whom Does an Adult Nurse Usually Work?

Adult nurses are the primary point of contact for adult patients and their families, and they play an essential role in professional and medical staff teams. They frequently collaborate with other professionals, such as physicians and healthcare assistants. Once certified, an adult nurse will work in a hospital or a community setting, such as a care home or a patient's home; this is becoming increasingly popular.

How Many Hours per Week Does a Nurse Work?

On average, adult nurses work 37.5 hours each week. In hospitals, shift work is performed, which involves regular unsocial hours (nights, early starts, evenings, weekends, and bank holidays). There is an expanding opportunity for 9 a.m. to 5 p.m. work in sectors other than the community, specialist units, and clinics, such as industry and commerce.

EXPECT THESE AS AN ADULT NURSE

As an adult nurse, you may occasionally face challenges and be presented with numerous possibilities to advance your profession. What to expect when working as an adult nurse is discussed in the sections that follow:

- Hours of work that are adaptable based on the shift you choose.
- When working in a hospital, an award, or a patient's home, the working conditions and setting vary frequently. Occasionally, you must care for a large number of patients in a ward or one or two patients in intensive care or a high dependency unit.
- There are numerous opportunities for professional breaks and retraining in a short amount of time, such as working abroad.
- You can work as a freelance consultant, which is possible through agencies as a private nurse or for senior nurses.

Did you Know?

A global survey by McKinsey & Company in 2022 found that between 28% and 38% of nurse respondents in the United States, the United Kingdom, Singapore, Japan, and France said they were likely to leave their current role in direct patient care in the next year.

Responsibilities of an Adult Nurse

Adult nursing is a dynamic field of work. A typical day at the office may be both tough and thrilling. Depending on your nursing function and specialty, your duties would also vary. As an adult nurse, you'll need to:

- assist doctors with examinations and decide what care to give.
- respond quickly to emergencies.
- write patient care plans.
- implement plans for tasks such as preparing patients for operations, treating wounds, and monitoring pulse, blood pressure, and temperature.
- observe and record the condition of patients.
- mentor student and junior nurses.
- supplying drips and blood transfusions.
- using specialist equipment.
- monitoring and recording patient progress.
- gain the trust and confidence of each patient.
- supporting patients and their relatives.

KEYWORD

Blood transfusion is the process of transferring blood products into a person's circulation intravenously.

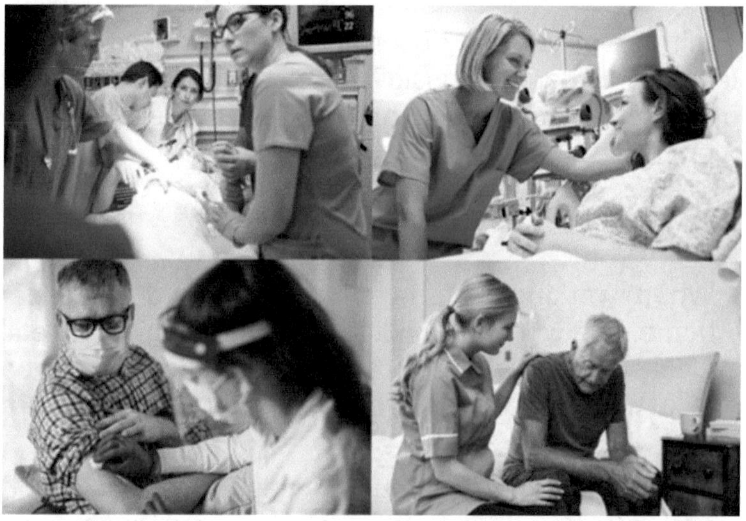

How Much Does an Adult Nurse Make?

The average registered nurse salary in the United Kingdom is £34,163 per year or £17.52 per hour. The good news is that 94% of nursing students find a job within six months of completing their degree (only 1% remain unemployed after six months).

NHS pay their staff when they work in an unsocial hour. Though in private sectors payments for the unsocial hour are not guaranteed, so you have to contact your employer before joining. The NHS nurses are entitled to a pension scheme, sickness, and maternity benefits. Salaries in London are much higher than in other areas of the UK. You'll be paid on the NHS Agenda for Change (AFC) pay system.

KEYWORD

Agenda for Change (AFC) allocates posts to set pay bands by giving consideration to aspects of the job, such as the skills involved, under an NHS Job Evaluation Scheme.

The Salary scales in NHS (National Health Services) for an adult nurse are:

- Freshly graduated and fully qualified nurse: £24,214 to £30,112 (Band 5 of the NHS Agenda for Change pay rates).
- An experienced nurse such as nurse team leader: £30,401 to £37,267 (Band 6).
- At more senior levels such as nurse advanced, modern matron, and nurse consultant: £37,570 to £72,597 (Bands 7 to 8c).

Who Are the Employers of Adult Nurses?

There are numerous options for adult nurses to work in intriguing disciplines, however, most of them are employed in hospital settings. Adult nurses work in hospitals, GP practices, the community (connected to a health clinic or general practice), residential homes, and hospices. However, geography is irrelevant when it comes to employing their expertise to meet the requirements of their patients.

When you are completely qualified and have sufficient experience, you can work as a nurse educator or provide health education in lieu of performing clinical work. Options include:

- Residential nursing homes
- Overseas aid and development
- Prisons
- Air ambulance services
- Community and school health education units
- Emergency helplines
- General practices
- Nursing agencies
- Occupational health
- Private healthcare organizations

- Schools and universities
- Specialist units and hospices
- The armed forces
- Voluntary organizations
- Health promotion
- Holiday companies
- Leisure cruise ships
- Research, teaching, and education

KEYWORD

Volunteering allows you to connect to your community and make it a better place.

ENROLMENT REQUIREMENTS TO STUDY IN ADULT NURSING

Grades and requirements vary between institutions. Always confirm the entry requirements for the particular university and course details before applying.

Certificates and Background Check

To study nursing in the UK, you'll usually need at least two A-Levels in either biology, chemistry, mathematics, physics, or psychology. You'll also need five GCSEs in grades C and above, including in English, math, and science. You will also have to:

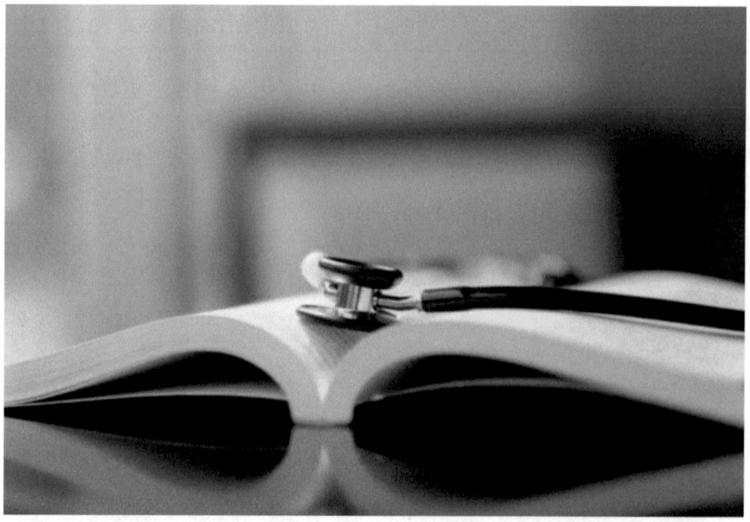

- Demonstrate evidence of literacy and numeracy.
- Complete a health questionnaire and identify any special needs related to a disability.

- You'll need to complete a DBS disclosure check (for criminal records) to ensure public protection and safety.
- Allow the university to check whether you have a police record. You will not automatically get rejected if you have a criminal conviction or caution. The university will take into account the circumstances and will treat any information in the strictest of confidence.

KEYWORD

Workforce is a concept referring to the pool of human beings either in employment or in unemployment.

Tips for Applying

Universities are seeking individuals who could become outstanding nurses in the future. Your course will likely entail hands-on experience with the general public. Try to demonstrate appropriate traits, such as communication and people skills, when applying for a course. Your application will benefit greatly from your work experience. This could be accomplished, for instance, through volunteering or collaborating with:

- NHS trust
- Private clinic
- Charities, such as St John Ambulance
- Care homes
- Daycare centers
- Youth organizations, such as scouts and guides

Qualification Required to Work as an Adult Nurse

The majority of applicants must earn a degree in (adult) nursing. In order to work as a nurse in the United Kingdom, you will require a full-time or part-time 3-year undergraduate degree. The undergraduate nursing programs for adults consist of Bachelor of Science in Nursing (BSN). You will have the opportunity to make a daily difference in the lives of people in each of these sectors. You will have the opportunity to make a daily difference in the lives of people in each of these sectors.

Many businesses increasingly favor nurses with a Bachelor of Science in Nursing (BSN) over an Associate of Science in Nursing (ASN) or Registered Nurse (RN) credential. Bachelor of Science in Nursing (BSN)-prepared nurses get the extensive knowledge and clinical experience necessary for success in today's complex health care system.

Nursing degrees are not solely based on book learning. The clinical practice portion of the program gives you direct experience dealing with patients and their families. You could be stationed at hospitals, the community, patients' homes, or independent groups, among others. The remaining time is devoted to intellectual pursuits. After graduating from the university, you must be registered with the Nursing & Midwifery Council (NMC).

KEYWORD

Domiciliary care services are provided in an individual's own home, whereas residential care involves the person moving permanently into a specialist supervised establishment set up solely to provide care.

ROLE OF NURSING IN ADULT SOCIAL CARE

The Covid-19 pandemic posed extraordinary difficulties for nurses working in adult social care, resulting in elevated levels of stress and anxiety, particularly in residences where a severe outbreak occurred. There are ongoing concerns regarding the lack of mental health and wellbeing support available.

Employers' Duties

Employers have a duty to:

- ensure that any nurses they employ as registered professionals meet all job requirements and can provide high standards of nursing care.
- conduct all checks required by their safe recruitment and selection procedures.
- respect the nurse's clinical autonomy and skills as a registered professional.
- support and facilitate their continuing professional development and revalidation.
- consider the skill mix required in their workforce to achieve the standards of care required.
- deploy their registered nurses to make the best use of their knowledge and skills in relation to those of others involved in meeting people's care and support needs.
- ensure they have the resources they need to carry out their roles effectively and efficiently.
- refer where necessary allegations or evidence of misconduct that breaches the professional code of practice to the NMC for investigation in addition to following other disciplinary procedures.
- be aware of ongoing emotional and practical challenges

as a consequence of the Covid-19 pandemic and be able to signpost them for appropriate support as necessary.

Employees' Duties

Registered nurses employed in a social care setting must:

- work in partnership with other careers and staff to achieve service standards and goals.
- use their professional judgment to achieve the required outcomes for service users.
- provide the necessary clinical leadership demanded of their role and responsibilities.
- take responsibility for their conduct, which should uphold their professional code of practice and values.
- ensure they provide safe person-centered nursing care by being responsive to people's needs and always acting in their best interests.
- keep up to date with best clinical practice and guidance.
- keep their registration requirements up to date.
- always be professional, and promote trust in their abilities and decision-making.
- communicate with and seek support from peers or manager regarding personal, professional, health issues or other concerns as a consequence of the Covid-19 pandemic.

Care Quality Commission Compliance

The Health and Social Care Act of 2008 establishes a unified regulatory framework for all health and care services in England that fall under its registration authority. This means that those receiving nursing care in their own homes, in care facilities, or in nursing homes can expect their service to be evaluated using the same criteria as hospitals and NHS primary care teams. Patients should expect safe, effective, kind, responsive, and well-led care regardless of where they are receiving nursing services.

Care providers with a nursing component will register for one or more regulated activities, such as:

- accommodation and nursing care (nursing home).
- nursing care (a service primarily led by registered nurses).

- treatment of disease, disorder, or injury (where, for example, qualified nurse is responsible for a program of care and treatment as in a residential intermediate care or rehabilitation unit or a reablement program carried out by a domiciliary care service).

KEYWORD

Social care services provide support to people with learning disabilities, physical disabilities/ilnesses and mental illnesses.

There are no specific requirements regarding nursing care, nursing homes, or the employment of registered nurses in the Health and Social Care Act 2008 (Regulated Activities) Regulations 2014. Regulation 18 "Staffing" suggests that where nurses are engaged as registered professionals, there must be enough of them to meet the needs of service users, and providers must meet their support and development needs as they do with all of their workers.

In practice, nursing facilities must have adequate registered nurses available 24 hours a day. The standards do not specify ratios or percentages, allowing providers some latitude in establishing the skill mix of their workforce.

CQC Inspections

Due to the coronavirus outbreak, routine CQC inspections of health and care services in England were suspended.

The CQC maintained its risk-based approach to inspection while taking measures to expand system capacity. They acknowledge that services continue to be under extraordinary pressure, putting safety and quality at risk. Recognizing the need for CQC as an organization to be responsive to the severe challenges various areas of the health and social care system are facing, their focus remains on helping services to provide safe treatment.

Infection Prevention and Control Inspections

The CQC have been undertaking specific infection prevention and control inspections (IPC) in care homes and continued to monitor this over the winter period.

CQC plan to provide further updates regarding the progress of their work, including Provider Collaboration Reviews, how they are returning to inspections and how they are assessing IPC when undertaking targeted and focused inspections. They are encouraging input to their Insight documents via their digital platform CitizenLab.

A New Strategy for the Changing World of Health and Social Care — CQC's Strategy from 2021

The CQC consulted with health and social care professionals, providers, and stakeholders on their proposed strategy for 2021 and beyond. They acknowledge the need for more flexibility in their approach and plan to change the way it regulates to help manage future risk and uncertainty.

Over 75% of respondents to the strategy consultation either "fully" or "mostly" supported proposals under each of the four themes in the strategy which are as follows:

- People and communities.
- Smarter regulation with assessments being more flexible and dynamic and updating of ratings more regularly.
- Safety through learning with stronger safety cultures and learning and improvement demonstrated.
- Accelerating improvement.

Wales Standards Compliance

Wales has required all care services to re-register with the Care Inspectorate Wales (CIW) in line with the requirements of the Regulation and Inspection of Social Care (Wales) Act 2016. Care homes are described in terms of care homes with care or care homes with nursing, which is a similar distinction to that taken in England.

The most recent Commencement Order in respect of the Act is: The Regulation and Inspection of Social Care (Wales) Act 2016 (Commencement No. 6, Savings and Transitional Provisions) Order 2019.

From 2 April 2018, this brought into effect the necessary provisions in Part 1 of the Act relating to the registration and regulation of care homes, secure accommodation, residential family centers and domiciliary support services in Wales.

Care Inspectorate Wales has published guidance for providers in respect of the registration of services under the Act.

Nurses Agencies are not covered by the Act, so do not require registration with the CIW. However, if a nursing service is being provided directly to people in their own homes, it must be registered as a domiciliary support service.

KEYWORD

Professional development is gaining new skills through continuing education and career training after entering the workforce.

The Regulated Services (Service Providers and Responsible Individuals) (Wales) Regulations 2017 require any form of nursing care to comply with the regulations generally, but specifically in relation to regulations:

KEYWORD

Primary care network is a structure which brings general practitioners together on an area basis, possibly with other clinicians, to address chronic disease management and prevention.

- ***Statement of Purpose***. The provision of nursing care should be described in the Statement of Purpose, particularly if the provider intends to provide nursing care as distinct from personal care only.
- ***Provider Assessment***. Nursing needs must be assessed by a registered nurse with the relevant skills.
- ***Staffing***. A home with nursing must ensure that it employs sufficient numbers of competent registered nurses, and where users require 24-hour nursing care, they must always have available sufficient nursing resources. Providers must show how they determine numbers and competency levels of the nursing staff needed.
- ***Supporting and Developing Staff***. Providers must enable registered nurses to keep up to date with their NMC registration status (through continuing professional development and revalidation).

Chief Nurse for Adult Social Care

The position of Chief Adult Social Care nurse, which was initially announced in September 2020 as part of the government's Covid-19 plan to provide clinical leadership for social care, has been made permanent.

Professor Deborah Sturdy OBE, the chief nurse for adult social care, expressed her desire to increase the number of registered nurses employed in the field. She emphasized that social care nursing is a highly skilled and sophisticated field of practice that provides advanced clinical decision-making, autonomy, care coordination, and leadership in difficult situations.

Enhanced Health in Care Homes

The NHS Long Term Plan included a commitment to roll out the *Framework for Enhanced Health in Care Homes (EHCH)* across England between 2020 and 2024.

EHCH moves towards proactive person-centered care focusing on individual service users' needs and those of their families and care home staff. This is via working across organizations in a more cohesive way so the service users will receive better, more coordinated care, delivered where they live, which enables:

- improved outcomes for service users via better management of their long-term condition/s.
- reduction in unplanned hospital admissions.
- reduction in hospitals as the place of death.

Elements of the EHCH were positioned quickly in May 2020 to support care home residents through the first wave of the Covid-19 pandemic. This interim service has transitioned to a more comprehensive service from 1 October 2020 and Primary Care Networks (PCNs) in collaboration with community healthcare providers became responsible for delivering the EHCH framework.

- Each care home being aligned to a named PCN and having a named clinical lead and weekly multidisciplinary team support.
- Support for care home residents with suspected or confirmed Covid-19 via remote monitoring and face-to-face assessment if deemed clinically appropriate.

Wider support included:

- pulse oximeters available to care homes that did not have the recommended number of devices, to help identify "silent hypoxia" and rapid deterioration of those with Covid-19.
- rehabilitation for those recovering from Covid-19, provided by both primary and community healthcare services.
- training and development for care home staff.
- support with data, IT, and technology, including access to care records and secure email.

The Care Provider Alliance has published a guide for care homes, which provides advice for managers on how to support their service users benefit from the service. It also provides information on how to work effectively with PCN clinical leads to ensure the health of service users is improved.

KEYWORD

Primary care network is a structure which brings general practitioners together on an area basis, possibly with other clinicians, to address chronic disease management and prevention.

Mental Health Challenges and Promoting Wellbeing for Nurses in Social Care during the Pandemic

Significant stress and mental health issues arose for social care nurses due to work-related pressures, high exposure to suffering, a lack of personnel, and inadequate support.

As the ongoing Covid-19 pandemic approaches the two-year mark, the situation continues to evolve. There are enduring concerns regarding the lack of mental health and wellbeing support available to the workforce. The CQC State of Health Care and Adult Social Care in England report stated that health and social care personnel are weary as a result of the pandemic, that the workforce is diminished, and that this has had a significant impact on care services as a whole.

The Chief Executive Officer of Care England also identified persistent nursing issues in the sector, as well as the impact of mandatory Covid vaccination, personnel shortages, and a lack of training opportunities, as pressures. Social Care Institute of Excellence (SCIE) and other sector organizations, such as Skills for Care, organized national forums and "meetup" events that were well-received by employees, and there is a request for national organizations to continue facilitating such groups formed during the epidemic.

Did you get it?

SCIE was commissioned by the Department of Health (now called the Department of Health and Social Care) to provide support over the Care Act 2014; looking at issues such as assessment and eligibility, safeguarding adults and advocacy.

Values and Principles of Nursing Care

Nursing values are enshrined in the NMC Code of Practice with which all nurses must comply to meet the terms of their registration. Updated in 2018 to include the new role of nurse assistants, which is being introduced in England, the code is divided into four main sections and several sub-sections. There is separate guidance for employers of registered nurses.

1. Prioritizing People

Nurses must be person-centered care in all aspects of their practice in line with the fundamental standards that apply to all health and social care services, i.e.:

- providing compassionate care that respects people's dignity and human rights
- listening to and empowering people to be fully involved in their own care and the decisions that must be made about it
- being responsive to people's needs and always acting in their best interests

- respecting people's needs for privacy and confidentiality

2. Practicing Effectively

In this section the code provides the building blocks of positive outcome-oriented nursing practice, emphasizing the importance of:

- evidence-based clinical judgments.
- clear communication with patients, service users and colleagues.
- sound recording and reporting.
- good teamwork and working relationships.
- sharing ideas, experiences and learning to promote continuous development and better care.

KEYWORD

Leadership is the ability of an individual or a group of people to influence and guide followers or members of an organization, society or team.

As registered professionals, nurses are responsible to themselves for their professional judgments, but many have leadership roles and powers of delegation. Therefore they could be accountable for work that they delegate to others, who are not in nursing roles.

As autonomous professionals, they must also be responsible for taking out indemnity insurance cover.

3. Preserve Safety

This section essentially addresses the nurse's duty of care to keep everyone they treat safe from harm. It requires nurses to:

- follow all safeguarding policies and procedures.
- always raise concerns about people's safety and risk of being harmed.
- ensure the safe administration of medicines for which they are responsible.
- prevent harm, for example, by assessing risks identifying and acting on possible mistakes, and learning from any that have been made.

4. Promote Professional and Trust

This section shows how the registered nurse must always be upholding the reputation of their profession by, for example:

- always acting honestly and within the law.
- never abusing their position in relation to their patients and service users by accepting large gifts or bribes.

- meeting their registration requirements through continuous professional development and revalidation.
- co-operating fully with audits and investigations (that might also test their duty of candour).
- being responsive to complaints and concerns.

Contributions of Registered Nurses to Social Care

KEYWORD

Social environment refers to the immediate physical and social setting in which people live or in which something happens or develops.

Registered nurses assist in the delivery of both residential and community social care. Skills for Care (2019) has compiled a summary of the contributions made by registered nurses employed in the adult social care sector as opposed to the NHS.

Registered nurses are employed mostly by independent health and care providers in nursing homes and community services.

Excluded from this number are those with a nursing degree who are employed in non-registered professional nursing positions, such as care workers or registered managers of care homes without nursing. Nursing skills are still applicable in these positions.

The report indicates that registered nurses contribute significantly to the well-being of service users by addressing their health care needs within a social environment.

In the broad social care industry, registered nurses occupy a variety of jobs, with many assuming both management and clinical responsibilities, which are typically executed in a leadership capacity. As accountable health professionals, they can be expected to be responsible for:

- assessment, evaluation and review of individual health needs.
- complex, evidence-based clinical decision making.
- planning and coordinating care plans.
- liaising with external stakeholders.
- creating a culture that supports compassion in care.
- appropriate delegation and supervision of assistant practitioners and care staff.

Their value to social care users and providers is also proven through their abilities to operate across health and social care boundaries, for example, in terms of:

- helping to avoid unnecessary hospital admissions.
- supporting early discharge.
- managing long term, complex and enduring conditions.
- preventing ill-health.
- managing convalescent and reablement care.
- promoting and leading health and wellbeing programs.

Remember

The nursing process is made up of five steps: 1. evaluate, 2. implement, 3. plan, 4. diagnose, and 5. assess. Nurses are able to use this process from the American Nurses Association to determine the best care they can provide for the patient.

Community Nursing Care Services

People residing in their own homes and in residential care facilities should have access to a variety of NHS services, such as community nursing. Domiciliary care services that register to provide nursing care with personal care or under the more specialized registration category "treatment of disease disorder or injury" may also provide nursing care services.

Typically, domiciliary care services that are registered to offer nursing care serve persons living in their own homes who have significant needs and disabilities, such as brain-injured individuals, and who require nursing expertise. Their care, or portions thereof, may be paid by the NHS and coordinated by the local Clinical Commissioning Group (CGC) in collaboration with the local government. In such cases, the majority of care may still be provided by care workers under nursing guidance and supervision.

The pandemic of coronavirus continues to have an effect on the provision of community nursing care services. Where GP access has been restricted in care homes, community nurses have encountered difficulties liaising with GPs, and for nurses working in social care, their tasks and abilities have expanded to match the rising complexity of service users' demands. Rapid use of technology has supported changes in work practices, such as virtual triage, difficult hospital discharges, and hospital admissions. Positive "virtual" communication with PCNs, GPs, and other health care experts has been enabled by technology. For many, the absence of a physically present team, especially when the delivery of care has been extremely distressing or difficult, has highlighted the need for ongoing support networks.

Care Homes with Nursing

Integrated health and social care are provided in a residential environment by nursing homes. According to statistics (from CQC,

Skills for Care, Social Care Wales, and the Competition and Marketing Authority), there are fewer nursing homes than care homes without nursing, although the number of nursing homeplaces is equivalent to the number of care homeplaces.

KEYWORD

Global Burden of Disease (GBD) provides a comprehensive picture of mortality and disability across countries, time, age, and sex.

This is because nursing homes are often larger than care homes and more likely to be operated by corporations. There are several very specialized nursing homes for younger folks, who frequently have complex needs due to chronic illnesses and/or impairments.

The Competition and Marketing Authority study of care homes for older people (2017) commented that 80% of care providers were running single homes accounting for just under 30% of places — these are too more likely to be care homes without nursing — while just 30 providers accounted for another 30% with the rest running more than one home. Nursing homes are more likely to be owned by multiple-home organizations.

In care facilities that do not offer a nursing service, community-based visiting nurses should fulfill nursing demands. For an individual paying for their own care, the decision to seek a place in a more expensive nursing home as opposed to a care home without nursing may be a matter of personal preference, with the reasons being less medical and more psychological, such as the individual feeling more secure knowing that nursing assistance is always available on the premises as opposed to having to be obtained on a visiting basis.

The NHS Long Term Plan

According to the most recent Global Burden of Disease (GBD) study, the top five causes of premature death in England are cardiovascular disease and stroke, cancer, respiratory disorders, dementia, and self-harm. The mortality rate attributable to heart and circulatory disorders in the United Kingdom has decreased by more than three-quarters during the past four decades; yet, cardiovascular disease remains the leading cause of premature death, and the rate of progress has slowed. These findings were utilized to build the NHS Long-Term Plan's priorities (2019).

NHS England stated that the growth in the average age of the population will necessarily result in an increase in the number of service users requiring a higher degree of support at home, in care and nursing homes, and in NHS care services.

The NHS Long-Term plan, which spans 10 years, includes the following areas pertaining exclusively to older adults:

- Additional years of life are not usually spent in good health, and people are likely to live with multimorbidities, frailty, or dementia; therefore, it is essential to enable older people to live well. Men aged over 2.4 years and women over three years have "substantial" care requirements.
- Care improvements for patients with dementia and delirium, regardless of whether they are hospitalized or at home. Over the past decade, the NHS has quadrupled the rate of dementia diagnosis and cut antipsychotic medicine prescriptions by half.
- Examining the effectiveness of social care services. The government has pledged to protect money for adult social care for the next five years to prevent the NHS from facing increased pressures.
- Pneumonia treatment is a big drain on NHS resources; therefore, enhancing how this is managed should assist to alleviate winter pressures.
- Why Caregivers will benefit from increased attention and support, and many caregivers are older individuals with complicated health requirements and many diseases. Such caregivers will be acknowledged, and extra support will be available to meet their unique health requirements.

Other areas include the following.

- Arrangements for integrated care to enable individuals to receive the appropriate care at the appropriate time and in the optimal care setting, with greater support for service users in residential care homes to attempt to minimize emergency hospital admissions. Provision of improved social care and community support to delay the onset of frailty, as well as restructuring of outpatient services. It has been reported that the requirements of nursing home residents are not always adequately assessed and met, resulting in unwarranted, unplanned, and avoidable hospitalizations.

KEYWORD

Pneumonia is an infection that affects one or both lungs. It causes the air sacs, or alveoli, of the lungs to fill up with fluid or pus. Bacteria, viruses, or fungi may cause pneumonia.

Regulation of Nursing Homes

Nursing homes, as defined by the Nursing Homes Registration Act of 1927, are "any facility utilized or planned to be used for the reception and provision of nursing care to persons suffering from any illness, injury, or infirmity." However, it wasn't until 1980 that nursing homes were legally obliged to be run by either a licensed physician or a registered nurse of the first degree.

From 1927 to the Care Standards Act of 2000, nursing facilities were inspected by health authorities; beginning in 1984, local government inspection teams also inspected residential care institutions. Under regulations enacted in 1984, nursing homes could also apply for "dual registration," or a combination of nursing and non-nursing beds. Inspectors from the health and local government inspected dual-registration residences together.

Remember

Residential care facilities or senior care facilities are small private facilities, usually with 20 or fewer residents (some might house as few as three or four people) that are staffed round the clock, delivering non-institutional home-based services to seniors who do not need 24-hour nursing care.

Under the Care Standards Act of 2000, the distinction between nursing and non-nursing care homes was eliminated, and care homes are now registered for personal and/or personal care and inspected according to a common standards framework (originally the national minimum care standards, now "fundamental standards").

Under the current registration system (Health and Social Care Act of 2008), nursing homes are certified to provide "accommodation with nursing care" while personal care facilities are registered to provide "accommodation with personal care." "Nursing care" includes "personal care".

A nursing home that provides specialized forms of care and treatment apart from conventional health care provision, such as intermediate care or rehabilitation programs, may also be required to register under "treatment of disease, condition, or injury."

Nursing and Non-Nursing Roles and Tasks

In a multi-purpose setting such as a nursing home, where the majority of direct care is provided by health care and care assistants and where residents have both social and health care needs, it can be difficult to distinguish between nursing and non-nursing duties and responsibilities. What constitutes a "nursing need" can often be hard to define. Much depends on the training and ability of the caregiver to perform certain jobs, as well as the skill mix of the entire team. The Nursing and Midwifery Council (NMC) outlines expectations of those on the register when they delegate to others. These requirements apply, irrespective of who the activity is being delegated to. This may be another registered professional, a non-registered colleague, or a patient or carers and RNs should:

- only delegate tasks and duties that are within the other person's scope of competence, making sure that they fully understand the instructions.
- make sure that everyone they delegate tasks to are adequately supervised and supported so they can provide safe and compassionate care.
- confirm that the outcome of any task delegated to someone else meets the required standard.

Nursing Tasks

The following lists the needs typically found in nursing homes in which the registered nurse plays a vital role in one or more respects because of their qualifications and expertise; not necessarily exclusively but often with other specialist help. The list is not exhaustive.

• Assessing mental and emotional health and wellbeing, and promoting healthy lifestyles.
• Continence promotion and management, including procuring and applying suitable aids, and, where necessary, carrying out specific clinical procedures such as manual bowel evacuation or use of irrigation systems.
• Dementia care, particularly where the person has multiple health needs. See Dementia Care topic
• Diabetes management, including supervising medication and injections, and training people to self-inject.
• End of life assessment and care planning.
• Falls prevention, including risk assessments and developing fall prevention and management plans.
• Hearing and sight.
• Infection prevention and control management.
• Initiation of emergency treatments such as in cases of anaphylactic shock, diabetic episodes, and epileptic seizures.
• Maintaining responsibility for clinical treatment rooms and their equipment and facilities, including diagnostic and monitoring equipment uses, and materials for routine procedures such as dressings.
• Management and safe use of specialist medical devices and equipment e.g. use of oxygen cylinders, suction machines.
• Management of stoma appliances and catheters.
• Medication administration and management, including anticipatory medicine needs and safe storage procedures.
• Nutrition and hydration, including screening and monitoring of people's nutritional and hydration provision.
• Oral and mouth care.

• Pain Management, particularly in palliative and end of life care.
• Resuscitation policies and procedures.
• Skin care, including prevention and treatment of skin damage, particularly pressure sores.
• Tracheostomy care.
• Wound care including wound assessment, applying wound care products and dressings, and training others in the procedures involved.

Changing Roles

The role of nursing is constantly changing, and new nursing models are being developed and introduced in specific areas, particularly dementia care. In these new models, nurses will be asked to provide clinical leadership for integrated health and social care teams providing service in a range of settings and places.

During the initial phase of the Covid-19 epidemic, nursing responsibilities were altered, and some nurses were redeployed to positions that required them to apply new or seldom-used abilities.

In the form of the Care Certificate and a uniform code of professional conduct, new health care assistants and social care professionals now share a common induction training framework. As frontline employees with adequate training, they can frequently obtain employment by migrating from one service setting to another.

Healthcare assistants can also be taught to do duties that were once considered nurse duties. Consequently, nursing duties have become both more diverse and specialized. In England, there are plans to introduce a new role of nursing associate, which is seen to be a level above that of health care assistant but below that of a registered nurse, though it will entail registering with the Nursing and Midwifery Council (NMC).

There is an increase in the usage of advanced nurse practitioners, who have the same level of clinical responsibility as a physician and can be found in both primary care and hospital settings. Additionally, nurses can be licensed to dispense medications. In hospitals, there is also the emergence of nurse-led units that operate in collaboration with medical professionals rather than as subordinates.

The nursing associate is now a legally recognized title, and the NMC regulates the role in England. This means that only those who are qualified and registered as nursing associates can be employed by practices. The Code must be followed by nursing assistants who are subject to regulatory obligations such as revalidation and fitness to practice. All nursing associates will operate as part of a team, however, they may work alone when visiting patients in their homes or the community. The nursing associate program offers a variety of paths to certification, including apprenticeship.

REVIEW QUESTIONS

1. What do you understand aboutadult nursing?
2. Explain the career overview of an adult nurse.
3. How many hours does an adult nurse work?
4. What are the responsibilities of an adult nurse?
5. What are the values and principles of nursing care?

MULTIPLE CHOICE QUESTIONS

1. You are the RN charge nurse on the medical surgical unit, and you are in charge of delegating assignments for the shift. Which of the following would be the most appropriate to delegate to the LPN/LVN?

a. A 25-year-old patient who requires IV antibiotic therapy, and needs a PICC line dressing change before administering the antibiotic.

b. A 72-year-old patient who requires Lasix 20mg IV push

c. A 50-year-old patient who is 3 days post op and requires a simple dressing change

d. A 45-year-old patient who is a newly diagnosed diabetic and requires discharge teaching

2. You are caring for a patient who is newly diagnosed with Congestive Heart Failure (CHF). Which statement by the patient would indicate that your patient teaching has been a success?

a. I will watch my salt intake and ensure that I do not exceed 4g or 4000mg per day in my diet

b. I will conduct a daily weight, keep a log of my daily weight, and report to my doctor immediately any weight gain of 3 or more pounds in one day

c. If I feel that I am urinating too frequently, I will not take my diuretic for a few days to help with the frequency of urination, after all, I don't want to fall getting out of bed so much at night

d. I will just smoke one half pack of cigarettes per day, as this is healthier than one pack

3. Which statement by the client receiving anticoagulation therapy with Coumadin would indicate a need for further teaching?

a. If I notice that I have a bruise that is three inches or bigger and continually gets larger, I will seek immediate medical help.

b. I will eat green leafy vegetables in moderation, as they are healthy, but can increase the thickness of my blood, potentially causing a clot.

c. I will keep all scheduled appointments for blood work because it is important to monitor my PT/ INR levels to ensure that my Coumadin dose is therapeutic

d. If I get a severe headache, worse than any other headache I have ever had in my life, I will take two aspirin, and take a nap, as that should help

4. Which of the following foods should a patient receiving Coumadin therapy be instructed to eat in moderation?

a. Spinach and other green leafy vegetables

b. Corn

c. Brown Rice

d. Lean Chicken Breast

5. A client receiving Lopressor 50mg IV should most importantly have which vital signs checked prior to administration?

a. Temperature

b. Respirations

c. Blood pressure, and heart rate

d. Pain

Answers to Multiple Choice Questions

1. (c) 2. (b) 3. (d) 4. (a) 5. (c)

REFERENCES

1. Care Homes Market Study (2017), Competition and Marketing Authority, available on the CMA website
2. Principles of Nursing Practice, Royal College of Nursing, available from the RCN website
3. Registered nurses: Recognising the responsibilities and contribution of registered nurses within social care. Skills for Care (2019), available on the Skills for Care website
4. Registration under the Health and Social Care Act 2008. The Scope of Registration. Care Quality Commission (20150, available on the CQC website
5. The Code: Professional Standards of Practice and Behaviour for Nurses, Midwives and Nursing Associates (October 2018), Nursing and Midwifery Council, available on the NMC website

6. The Code. Professional Staff, Quality Services (Employers Guide), (NMC Updated 2018), available on the NMC website
7. The State of the Adult Social Care Sector and Workforce in England: 2018, Skills for Care (2018), available on the Skills for Care website
8. The Size and Structure of the Adult Social Care Workforce in England, Skills for Care, available on the Skills for Care website
9. The State of Healthcare and Adult Social Care in England 2017/18, Care Quality Commission, available on the CQC website
10. Workforce Intelligence Summary. Care Homes with Nursing in the Adult Care Sector 2018/19, Skills for Care (2018), available on the Skills for Care website
11. Employers' Responsibilities (2019), available on the NMC website
12. NHS Long Term Plan (2019), available on the NHS website
13. Making the Most of Student Nurse Placements (2021), available on the Skills for Care website
14. A New Strategy for the Changing World of Health and Social Care, Our Strategy from 2021, Care Quality Commission, available on the CQC website
15. Enhanced Health in Care Homes: A Guide for Care Homes (2021), The Care Provider Alliance, available on The Care Provider Alliance website

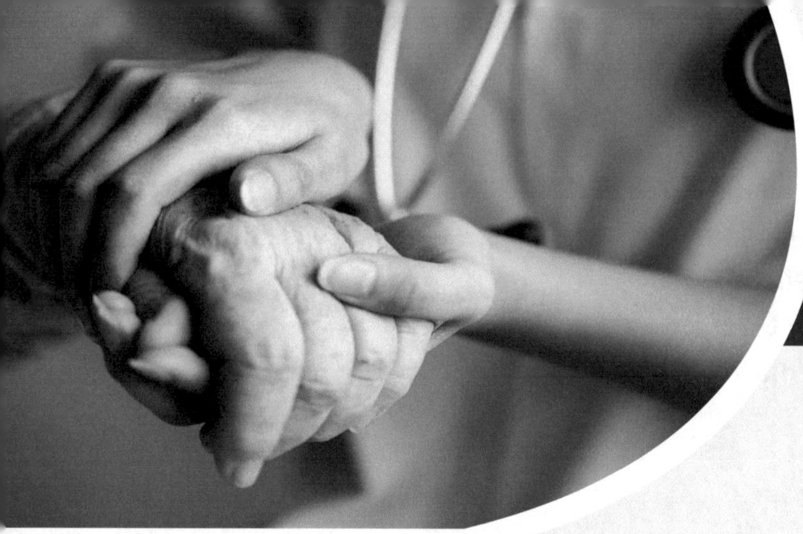

CHAPTER 6

GERONTOLOGICAL NURSING

"Every nurse was drawn to nursing because of a desire to care, to serve, or to help."

—Christina Feist-Heilmeier, RN

INTRODUCTION

Aging, the normal process of time-related change, begins with birth and continues throughout life. The U.S. Census Bureau forecasts that by 2030, there will be more individuals aged 65 or older than individuals aged 18 or younger. As the elderly population grows, so will the number of persons who reach extreme old age. It will be a challenge for health experts to develop measures to combat the increased prevalence of disease in this aging population. Numerous chronic illnesses prevalent in the elderly can be controlled, minimized, and even prevented. If adequate community-based support services are provided, it is more probable that seniors will maintain good health and functional independence.

Learning Objectives

After completing the chapter, you will be able to accomplish the following:

- History of gerontological nursing
- Attitude towards aging and older adults
- Definitions of gerontological nursing

- Concept and scope of gerontological nursing
- Principles of gerontological nursing
- Assessment of an elderly patient
- Approach to an elderly patient
- Levels of geriatric care and the role of a nurse
- Overview of geriatric care

Key-Terms

- Chronic health disorders
- Gerontic nurse
- Geriatric nurse
- Dyspnoea memory problems,
- Incontinence
- Gait disturbance
- Constipation
- Dizziness
- Rheumatic fever
- Poliomyelitis
- Polypharmacy
- Elder care management

HISTORY OF GERONTOLOGICAL NURSING

The history and development of gerontological nursing is rich in diversity and experiences, as is the population it serves. There has never been a better moment to be a gerontological nurse than now. Regardless of where they practice, nurses will at some point in their careers provide care for elderly persons. The health care movement is continually growing life expectancy; consequently, nurses must anticipate caring for a greater proportion of elderly patients in the coming decades. In light of the growing prevalence of acute and chronic health disorders among the elderly, nurses are in a crucial position to provide illness prevention and health promotion, as well as to promote healthy aging.

The American Journal of Nursing, the American Nurses Association (ANA), and the John A. Hartford Foundation Institute of Geriatric Nursing at New York University have made substantial contributions to the creation of gerontological nursing as a specialty. In the early 1960s, when the ANA recommended a specialist group for geriatric nurses and the founding of a geriatric nursing division, and hosted the first national nursing symposium on geriatric nursing practice, the specialty was formally acknowledged. Over the next three decades, the specialty's expansion exploded. The ANA Standards for Geriatric Practice and the Journal of Gerontological Nursing were initially published in the early 1970s (in 1970 and 1975, respectively). Following the implementation of federal programs such as Medicare and Medicaid, the health care market for seniors expanded rapidly. In the 1970s, the Veterans Administration supported a number of Geriatric Research Education and Clinical Centers (GRECCs) at VA medical facilities in the United States.

Through the construction of GRECCs, nurses were provided with extensive educational opportunities to learn about the care of older veterans. Additionally, the Kellogg Foundation supported a number of certificate nurse practitioner programs at colleges of nursing that prepared nurses to become geriatric nurse practitioners. These were not master's-level nursing schools, but they did supply geriatrics-trained nurses to suit the demands of an aging population. The terms geriatric nurse, gerontic nurse, and gerontological nurse have been used to designate nurses who care for the elderly. These terminologies have different connotations, but gerontological nursing gives a comprehensive perspective on the care of older persons. In 1976, the ANA Geriatric Nursing Division became the Gerontological Nursing Division and produced the Standards for Gerontological

Did you get it?

ICN was founded in 1899 by nursing organizations from Great Britain, the ANA for the United States, and Germany as charter members. The first ever ICN Congress was held in Buffalo New York in 1901. The next congress to take place in the United States was the Ninth ICN Quadrennial Congress in 1947, hosted by the ANA, at Atlantic City.

Nursing (Ebersole &Touhy, 2006; Meiner &Lueckenotte, 2006). The establishment of the National Gerontological Nursing Association and the American Nurses Association's (ANA) statement on the Scope and Standards of Gerontological Nursing Practice led to a major expansion of gerontological nursing during the 1980s. Increased numbers of nurses began to earn master's and doctoral degrees in gerontology, and institutions of higher learning launched programs to prepare nurses for advanced practice nursing in the subject (geriatric nurse practitioners and gerontological clinical nurse specialists).

TIPS

Geriatric care management is the process of planning and coordinating care of the elderly and others with physical and/or mental impairments to meet their long term care needs, improve their quality of life, and maintain their independence for as long as possible.

As a result, nurses began to explore gerontological nursing research as a field of study and interest in theories to develop nursing as a science emerged. Implementation of five Robert Wood Johnson (RWJ) Foundation Teaching Nursing Homes afforded nursing faculty and nursing homes the opportunity to collaborate in order to improve institutionalized elder care. An additional eight community-based RWJ grant–funded demonstration projects enabled older adults to remain in their homes and fostered cooperation between social service and health care agencies to partner in providing in-home care.

The NYU Division of Nursing founded the John A. Hartford Foundation Institute for Geriatric Nursing in the 1990s. It created an extraordinary impetus for enhancing nursing education and practice and expanding nursing research in the care of older individuals. Moreover, it emphasized geriatric public policy and consumer education. The Nurses Improving Treatment for Health system Elders (NICHE) initiative established a national reputation as the standard for acute care for elderly patients. Gerontological care has had a renaissance in the 21st century, as older persons receive full social standing and acknowledgment. As the baby boomer generation enters the elderly age bracket in 2011, these individuals will not only anticipate but also demand superior geriatric care. The Hartford Geriatric Nursing Initiative (HGNI) was created in 2003 via the joint efforts of the John A. Hartford Institute for Geriatric Nursing, the American Academy of Nursing, and the American Association of Colleges of Nursing (AACN). This effort significantly boosted the number of gerontological nurse scientists and the development of gerontological nursing practice based on scientific evidence. Multiple professional publications, books, websites, and organizations are currently devoted to the nursing care of elderly individuals. In 2008, the Journal of Gerontological Nursing Research emerged as one of the newest journals.

Numerous nursing pioneers are credited with the evolution of gerontological nursing as a subspecialty. The bulk of these nurses were from the United States, although two pioneers were from the United Kingdom. Florence Nightingale and Doreen Norton were pioneers in the field of geriatric care. Nightingale was the first true geriatric nurse because she accepted the role of nurse supervisor at an English institution analogous to our modern nursing homes. She cared after affluent women's maids and servants at the Care of Sick Gentlewomen in Difficult Circumstances Institution (Wykle& McDonald, 1997). Doreen Norton summarized her opinions on geriatric nursing in a 1956 address at the Student Nurses Association's annual conference in London. Later in her career, she specialized in elderly care and frequently wrote about the distinct and specific requirements of the elderly and the nurses caring for them. She identified the advantages of learning geriatric care in basic nursing education as:

- Learning patience, tolerance, understanding, and basic nursing skills.
- Witnessing the terminal stages of disease and the importance of skilled nursing care at that time.
- Preparing for the future, because no matter where one works in nursing the aged will be a great part of the care.
- Recognizing the importance of appropriate rehabilitation, which calls upon all the skills that nurses possess.
- Being aware of the need to undertake research in geriatric nursing (Norton, 1956).

KEYWORD

Nurse education consists of the theoretical and practical training provided to nurses with the purpose to prepare them for their duties as nursing care professionals.

ATTITUDE TOWARDS AGING AND OLDER ADULTS

As a professional in geriatric care, you may have preconceived notions about senior care. These notions are impacted by your observations of family members, friends, neighbors, the media, and older folks, as well as your personal experience with them. You may have a close relationship with your grandparents or have witnessed the aging of your parents. When you look in the mirror, the aging process may have been apparent to some of you. Whether or not we have taken the time to consciously consider it, this universal phenomenon known as aging has some significance for each of us.

Your perspective on aging and older folks is frequently influenced by your environment and the experiences you have had. Poor views toward aging or older persons (ageism) are commonly rooted in negative prior experiences. Many of our beliefs and assumptions about older folks may be unfounded. Some of you may already be familiar with ageism, which manifests itself similarly to sexism and racism through attitudes and acts. To investigate myths and realities, to distinguish fact from fiction, and to get an appreciation for what older persons have to offer is one rationale for researching the aging process.

The majority of your careers as geriatric health professionals will include caring for older persons, according to population figures. As Mathy Mezey, director of the John A. Hartford Foundation Institute for Geriatric Nursing at NYU, stated, —"The population of older Americans is exploding. Geriatric patients are not a subset of patients, but rather the focus of healthcare systems. High-quality care for the elderly involves an understanding of the complexities of the aging process and the various syndromes and diseases that might accompany aging".

KEYWORD

Gerontological nursing is an evidence-based nursing specialty that addresses the unique physiological, social, psychological, developmental, economic, cultural, spiritual, and advocacy needs of older adults

Perhaps you already have a positive attitude on providing care for the elderly. Consider devoting your time and energy to the practice of gerontological nursing, building on this principle. If, on the other hand, you are reading this chapter with the notion that gerontological nursing is a less desirable field of nursing, that only professionals who cannot find jobs elsewhere work in nursing homes, or that working with older people would be a last resort, you may need to reevaluate your beliefs. With knowledge of the facts and positive interactions with older individuals, you may change your mind.

Advocates for older persons, such as Nobel laureate Elie Wiesel, believe that older adults should be valued and revered as the keepers of our collective memory. As the keynote convention speaker for the American Psychological Association in 1997, Wiesel stated, an aged person represents wisdom and the possibility of a complete life. The worst curse is to make him or her feel useless.

As baby boomers (those born between 1946 and 1964) reach retirement age, the aging population is undergoing a tremendous shift. Because this phenomenon is occurring in numerous locations around the world, gerontology is where it's at! Providing care for the greatest number of elderly individuals in history will bring immense opportunity. The complexity of care for so many people with multiple physical and psychosocial problems will be a challenge for the most courageous nurses due to the rapid growth of the over-85 age group.

DEFINITIONS OF GERONTOLOGICAL NURSING

Gerontology is the umbrella word for the study of aging and/or the elderly. This includes the psychological and biosocial aspects of aging. Geriatrics, social gerontology, geropsychology, geropharmacology, financial gerontology, gerontological nursing, and gerontological rehabilitation nursing are all subfields of gerontology.

KEYWORD

Social gerontology is a multi-disciplinary sub-field that specializes in studying or working with older adults.

Geriatrics is commonly used as an umbrella term for the elderly, however, it primarily relates to the medical care of the elderly. As a result, numerous nursing publications and textbooks prefer the term gerontological nursing over geriatric nursing.

Social gerontology focuses primarily on the social elements of aging, as opposed to the medical or psychological components. Social gerontologists not only rely on research from all social disciplines — sociology, psychology, economics, and political science — they also aim to comprehend how biological processes of aging influence the social elements of aging.

Geropsychology is a subfield of psychology concerned with assisting older individuals and their families to preserve health, overcome obstacles, and realize their full potential as they age.

Geropharmacology is the study of pharmacology as it pertains to senior citizens. CGP is the credential for a geropharmacology-certified pharmacist (certified geriatric pharmacist).

Another developing discipline, financial gerontology combines knowledge of financial planning and services with specialized knowledge of the requirements of older persons. Financial gerontology is defined by Cutler (2004) as "the intellectual junction of two fields, gerontology and finance, with practitioner and academic components in both."

Gerontological rehabilitation nursing blends knowledge of gerontological nursing with principles and practices of rehabilitation. In gerontological rehabilitation, nurses frequently provide care to elderly patients with chronic illnesses and long-term functional restrictions, such as stroke, head injury, multiple sclerosis, Parkinson's disease, spinal cord injury, arthritis, joint replacements, and amputations. Gerontological rehabilitation nursing aims to assist older persons in regaining and maintaining the best level of function and independence possible, while preventing problems and improving quality of life.

Therefore, gerontological nursing falls within the nursing discipline and the scope of nursing practice. It requires nurses to advocate for the health of the elderly at all levels of disease prevention. Gerontological nurses work with healthy seniors in their communities, seniors with acute illnesses needing hospitalization and treatment, and seniors with chronic illnesses or disabilities in long-term care facilities, skilled care, home care, and hospice.

TIPS

The gerontological nursing scope of practice encompasses all older persons from "old age" till death.

CONCEPT AND SCOPE OF GERONTOLOGICAL NURSING

Gerontological nursing is informed by knowledge of the various elements that influence the health of older persons. Older persons are more likely than younger adults to suffer from at least one chronic health problem, such as diabetes, cardiovascular disease, cancer, arthritis, hearing loss, or Alzheimer's disease. In addition, drug metabolism alters with age, adding to the complexity of health care requirements.

Gerontological nurses work in numerous settings, including acute care hospitals, rehabilitation, nursing homes (also known as long-term care homes and skilled nursing facilities), assisted living facilities, retirement homes, community health organizations, and the patient's home. Depending on the geriatric's health, the sort of facility in which they should reside is determined. Assisted living facilities are also known as retirement homes for seniors since they provide care based on health issues. A skilled nursing facility, sometimes known as a nursing home, is a residence where residents get 24-hour care.

Gerontological nursing specialists have referred to older individuals as "the heart of healthcare." Due to the aging of the population and the complexity of the health care needs of some older folks, older adults are more likely to utilize health care services than younger ones. In many situations, older individuals constitute the bulk of patients. Experts urge, therefore, that all nurses, not just geriatric nurses, should have specialist expertise of older persons. This position was backed by 55 nursing specialty organizations in the United States.

PRINCIPLES OF GERONTOLOGICAL NURSING

According to Stanford School of Medicine- Ethno geriatrics, the principles of geriatric care include:

- Biopsychosocial approach: the integration of consideration of physical, psychological, and social factors in providing health care
- Use of multidisciplinary teams
- Importance of chronic illnesses and geriatric syndromes
- Importance of showing respect to older patients
- Goal of maximizing function Awareness and sensitivity to sensory changes
- Age-appropriate dosing and avoidance of interactions of multiple medications
- Continuity of care through the different components of geriatric care
    - Geriatric primary care
    - Geriatric acute care
    - Geriatric rehabilitation
    - Geriatric long-term care
- Community based
    - Home care
    - Adult day care/day health care
    - Respite care
- Residential Services
    - Assisted living, board & care, adult care, or residential care
    - Nursing homes
    - Combinations of levels of care—Continuing care retirement communities
- Geriatric managed care: integration of primary, acute, and long-term care
    - Program of All-inclusive Care for the Elderly (PACE)

Did you get it?

A geriatric nursing specialty group was formed by the American Nurses Association in 1966, with the name changed to the Gerontological Nursing Division in 1976.

- U.S. Department of Veterans Affairs geriatric programs

According to Emory, the basic principles of gerontological nursing are:

Principles	Descriptions
1. Aging is not a disease	➢ Aging occurs at different rates between individuals, within individuals in different organ systems. ➢ Aging alone does not generally cause symptoms. ➢ Aging increases susceptibility to many diseases and conditions ("homeostenosis"). ➢ Aging people are heterogeneous-some are very healthy, some are very ill.
2. Medical conditions in geriatric patients are commonly chronic, multiple, and multifactorial	➢ Older individuals commonly suffer multiple chronic conditions, making management complex and challenging. ➢ Acute illness are superimposed on chronic conditions and their management. ➢ Treatment for one chronic or acute illness can influence the management of other underlying conditions. ➢ Multiple factors are generally involved in the pathogenesis of geriatric conditions.
3. Reversible and treatable conditions are often under-diagnosed and under-treated in geriatric patients	➢ Older individuals, caregivers, and health professionals mistakenly attribute symptoms to "old age". ➢ Many conditions present atypically in the geriatric population. ➢ Systematic screening for common geriatric conditions can help avoid undiagnosed, treatable conditions ➢ Geriatric "syndromes" are commonly undiagnosed and therefore not managed optimally, such as: delirium, gait, instability and falls, urinary incontinence, pain, and malnutrition.

4. Functional ability and quality of life are critical outcomes in the geriatric population	➢ Functional capacity, in combination with social supports, is critical in determining living situation and overall quality of life. ➢ Small changes in functional capability (e.g., the ability to transfer) can make a critical difference for quality of life of older patients and their caregivers. ➢ Standard tools can be used to measure basic and instrumental activities of daily living and overall quality of life.
5. Social history, social support, and patient preferences are essential aspects of managing geriatric patients	➢ Understanding the patient's life history and preferences for care are critical (place of birth, education, occupation, family relationships, spirituality, resources, willingness to take risks and utilize resources for care, etc). ➢ Living circumstances are critical to managing frail older patients. ➢ Caregiver availability, health, and resources are critical determinants of care planning for frail older patients.
6. Geriatric care is multidisciplinary	➢ Interdisciplinary respect, collaboration, and communication are essential in the care of geriatric patients and their caregivers. ➢ Various disciplines play an important role in geriatric care, e.g. nursing, rehabilitation therapists, dieticians, pharmacists, social workers, etc.
7. Cognitive and affective disorders are prevalent and commonly undiagnosed at early stages	➢ Aging is associated with changes in cognitive function. ➢ Common causes of cognitive impairment include delirium, Alzheimer's disease, and multi-infarct dementia. ➢ Geriatric depression is often undiagnosed. ➢ Screening tools for delirium, dementia, and depression should be used routinely.
8. Iatrogenic illnesses are common and many are preventable	➢ Polypharmacy, adverse drug reactions, drug-disease interactions, drug-drug interactions, inappropriate medications all common. ➢ Complications of hospitalization, such as falls, immobility, and deconditioning can be serious and life-threatening.

9. Geriatric care is provided in a variety of settings ranging from the home to long-term care institutions	➢ There are specific definitions and criteria for admission to different types of care settings. ➢ Funding for care in different settings varies and depends on many factors. ➢ Transitions between care settings must be coordinated in order to avoid unnecessary duplication, medical errors, and patient injuries. ➢ Integrated, multi-level systems provide the most coordinated care for complex geriatric patients.
10. Ethical issues and end-of-life care are critical aspects of the practice of geriatrics	➢ Ethical issues arise almost every day in geriatric care. ➢ Advance directives are critical for preventing some ethical dilemmas. ➢ Principles of palliative care and end-of-life care are essential for high quality geriatric care.

ASSESSMENT OF AN ELDERLY PATIENT

- Frequently, additional time is required to interview and evaluate older patients, in part due to the fact that they may possess features that impede the examination. The following should be taken into account:
- ***Sensory deficits:*** Dentures, eyeglasses, or hearing aids, if regularly worn, should be worn throughout the interview to enhance communication. Also helpful are adequate illumination and the avoidance of visual or auditory distractions.
- ***Underreporting of symptoms:*** Elderly patients may not report symptoms they perceive to be a normal part of aging (e.g., dyspnoea, hearing or vision deficits, memory problems, incontinence, gait disturbance, constipation, dizziness, and falls). However, no symptom should be assigned to natural aging until a complete evaluation has been performed and all other potential reasons have been ruled out.
- ***Unusual manifestations of a disorder:*** In the elderly, typical manifestations of a disorder may be absent. Instead,

KEYWORD

Constipation is a condition in which a person has uncomfortable or infrequent bowel movements.

elderly patients may exhibit vague symptoms (e.g., fatigue, confusion, weight loss).

- ***Functional decline as the only manifestation:*** Disorders may only manifest as a reduction in function. In such situations, standard questions may be inappropriate. Patients with severe arthritis may not report pain, edema, or stiffness when questioned about joint symptoms, but if asked about changes in activities, they may state that they no longer take walks or volunteer at the hospital. Questions regarding the duration of functional decline (e.g., "How long have you been unable to do your own shopping?") can yield valuable information. Identifying individuals when they have just begun to struggle with basic or instrumental activities of daily living (BADLs or IADLs) may afford more opportunities for interventions to restore functions or prevent future decline, so preserving independence.
- ***Difficulty recalling:*** Patients may not accurately recall past illnesses, hospitalizations, operations, and drug usage; practitioners may be required to gather this information from another source (e.g., from family members, a home health aide, or medical records).
- ***Fear:*** The elderly may be hesitant to disclose symptoms because they connect hospitalization with death.
- ***Age-related disorders and problems:*** Depression (common among older who are vulnerable and ill), the cumulative losses of old age, and discomfort caused by a disorder may make the elderly less likely to supply clinicians with health-related information. Patients with impaired cognition may have trouble explaining their symptoms, making evaluation more difficult.

KEYWORD

Medical record are used somewhat interchangeably to describe the systematic documentation of a single patient's medical history and care across time within one particular health care provider's jurisdiction.

Interview

A clinician's knowledge of an elderly patient's everyday concerns, social circumstances, mental function, emotional state, and sense of well-being helps orient and guide the interview. Asking patients to describe a typical day elicits information regarding their mental and physical health. This strategy is especially effective during the initial encounter. Patients should be provided the opportunity to discuss matters of personal significance. Additionally, clinicians should inquire if patients have specific worries, such as a fear of falling. The resulting rapport can improve the clinician's ability to communicate with patients and their families.

In order to assess the patient's dependability, it may be required to conduct a mental status examination early in the interview; this examination should be conducted with tact so that the patient does not become embarrassed, insulted, or defensive. Beginning at age 70, screenings for physical and psychological issues should be performed annually.

Often, verbal and nonverbal clues (e.g., the way the story is told, tempo of speech, tone of voice, eye contact) can provide information, as for the following:

- ***Depression***: Elderly patients may omit or deny symptoms of anxiety or depression but betray them by a lowered voice, subdued enthusiasm, or even tears.
- ***Physical and mental health***: What patients say about sleep and appetite may be revealing.
- ***Weight gain or loss***: Clinicians should note any change in the fit of clothing or dentures.

A patient should be interviewed alone to facilitate the sharing of personal things, unless their mental state is impaired. Clinicians may also need to consult with a relative or caretaker, who frequently provides a unique viewpoint on the patient's mental and emotional health, as well as their level of function. These interviews may be conducted with or without the patient present.

Remember

If indicated, clinicians should consider the possibility of drug abuse by the patient and patient abuse by the caregiver.

The clinician should solicit the patient's consent before inviting a family member or caregiver, and should clarify that such conversations are standard procedure. If only the caregiver is being interviewed, the patient should be kept engaged (e.g., filling out a standardized assessment questionnaire, being interviewed by another member of the interdisciplinary team).

Medical History

When interviewing patients about their past medical history, clinicians should inquire about once-common illnesses (e.g., rheumatic fever, poliomyelitis) and outmoded therapies (eg, pneumothorax therapy for TB, mercury for syphilis). Immunization history (e.g., tetanus, influenza, pneumococcal), adverse reactions to vaccines, and tuberculosis skin test results are required. Clinicians should ask questions meant to methodically assess each body part or system (review of systems) in order to identify unmentioned illnesses and frequent complaints.

Drug History

The drug history should be recorded, and a copy should be given to patients or their caregiver. It should contain:

- Drugs used
- Dose
- Dosing schedule
- Prescriber
- Reason for prescribing the drugs
- Precise nature of any drug allergies

All drugs used should be recorded, including:

- Topical drugs (which may be absorbed systemically)
- OTC drugs (which can have serious consequences if overused and may interact with prescription drugs)
- Dietary supplements
- Medicinal herb preparations (because many can interact adversely with prescription and OTC drugs)

At the initial visit and occasionally thereafter, patients or their families should be requested to bring in all of the above medications and supplements. Clinicians can ensure that patients have the prescribed medications, but this does not guarantee adherence. It may be required to count the tablet numbers in each vial at the initial and subsequent visits. If a person other than the patient provides the medication, that individual is interrogated.

Patients should be asked to demonstrate their capacity to read (often small) labels, open (particularly child-resistant) containers, and identify medications. Patients should not combine their medications in a single container.

KEYWORD

Medicinal herbs have been discovered and used in traditional medicine practices since prehistoric times.

Alcohol, Tobacco, and Recreational Drug Use History

Patients who smoke should be urged to quit, and if they choose to continue, they should refrain from smoking in bed, as the elderly are more prone to fall asleep while doing so.

The elderly should be examined for symptoms of alcohol use disorders, which are underdiagnosed. These symptoms include bewilderment, irritability, aggressiveness, alcohol-related breath odor, decreased balance and gait, tremors, peripheral neuropathy, and nutritional deficits. Alcohol screening questionnaires including inquiries regarding the amount and frequency of alcohol usage can be beneficial. The 4 CAGE questions are brief and direct; the clinician asks the patient if they have ever felt:

KEYWORD

Dietary fiber or roughage is the portion of plant-derived food that cannot be completely broken down by human digestive enzymes.

- The need to cut down drinking.
- Annoyed by criticism about drinking.
- Guilty about drinking.
- The need for a morning “eye-opener”.

Two or more positive responses to the CAGE questions suggest the possibility of alcohol abuse. Questions about the use of other recreational drugs or substances of abuse also are appropriate.

Nutrition History

The type, quantity, and frequency of food eaten are determined. Patients who eat ≤ 2 meals a day are at risk of under nutrition. Clinicians should ask about the following:

- Any special diets (e.g., low-salt, low-carbohydrate) or self-prescribed fat diets
- Intake of dietary fiber and prescribed or OTC vitamins
- Weight loss and change of fit in clothing
- AThe money patients have to spend on food
- Accessibility to food stores and suitable kitchen facilities
- Variety and freshness of foods

The ability to eat (such as chewing and swallowing) is assessed. It may be hindered by xerostomia and/or dental issues, which are prevalent among the elderly. Decreased taste or fragrance may diminish the pleasure of eating, causing patients to consume less food. Patients with impaired vision, arthritis, immobility, or tremors may have trouble preparing meals and may damage themselves by burning themselves while cooking. Patients who are concerned about urine incontinence may decrease their hydration intake and, consequently, their food consumption.

Mental Health History

Mental health issues may be difficult to detect in elderly persons. Insomnia, changes in sleep patterns, constipation, cognitive impairment, anorexia, weight loss, exhaustion, obsession with physiological functions, and increased alcohol intake may have an alternative explanation in the elderly. Depression may be indicated by feelings of melancholy, hopelessness, and sobbing spells. The major affective symptom of depression may be irritability, while patients may have cognitive impairment. Generalized anxiety is the most prevalent mental condition in the elderly and is frequently accompanied by depressive symptoms.

Remember

Melancholy can have causes that aren't due to underlying disease. Examples include seeing a sad movie, loss of a loved one or object or a good thing coming to an end.

Patients should be questioned regarding delusions and hallucinations, previous mental health care (including psychotherapy, hospitalization, and electroconvulsive therapy), psychoactive drug use, and recent life changes. Several factors (e.g., recent loss of a loved one, hearing impairment, change in location or living situation, loss of independence) may lead to depression.

The spiritual and theological preferences of patients, including their personal interpretations of aging, deteriorating health, and death, must be understood.

Functional Status

As part of a full geriatric evaluation, it is decided if patients can function independently, require some assistance with basic activities of daily living (BADLs) or instrumental activities of daily living (IADLs), or require entire assistance. Patients may be asked open-ended questions about their capacity to perform activities, or they may be asked to complete a structured assessment instrument with questions about certain ADLs and IADLs.

Social History

Clinicians should acquire information on patients' living arrangements, including where and with whom they reside (e.g., alone in an isolated house, in a crowded apartment complex), the accessibility of their residence (e.g., stairs or a hill), and the available forms of transportation. These factors affect the ability of the elderly to acquire food, medical care, and other vital resources. Although difficult to schedule, a house visit can provide vital information. Clinicians can glean information about nutrition from the refrigerator's contents and about several ADLs from the condition of the lavatory. The number of rooms, the quantity and kind of phones, the existence of smoke and carbon monoxide detectors, the quality of the plumbing and heating system, and the presence of elevators, stairs, and air conditioning are determined. Home safety evaluations can detect potential fall hazards (e.g., insufficient illumination, slippery bathtubs, unanchored rugs) and offer fixes.

KEYWORD

Sexually transmitted diseases (STDs) are infections that are primarily transmitted through sexual contact. These infections can be caused by bacteria, viruses, parasites, or other microorganisms.

A patient's description of a typical day, including reading, television viewing, work, exercise, hobbies, and social interactions, provides useful information.

Clinicians should ask about the following:

- Frequency and nature of social contacts (e.g., friends, senior citizens' groups), family visits, and religious or spiritual participation)
- Driving and availability of other forms of transportation
- Caregivers and support systems (e.g., church, senior citizens' groups, friends, neighbors) that are available to the patient
- The ability of family members to help the patient (e.g., their employment status, their health, traveling time to the patient's home)
- The patient's attitude toward family members and their attitude toward the patient (including their level of interest in helping and willingness to help)

Patients' marital status is documented. Questions regarding sexual practices and satisfaction must be delicate, courteous, and thorough. The number and gender of sexual partners are identified, as well as the risk of sexually transmitted diseases (STDs). Many sexually active older adults are unaware of the rising frequency of sexually transmitted diseases (STDs) within their age group and do not follow or even know about safe sex practices.

Patients should be queried about their level of education, occupations, known exposures to radiation or asbestos, and current and former hobbies. It is described how retirement, a fixed income, or the death of a spouse or partner might cause financial issues. Financial or health issues may lead to the loss of one's home, social standing, or independence. Patients should be asked about previous ties with physicians; a long-standing relationship with a physician may have ended due to the physician's retirement, death, or the patient's relocation.

Advance Directives

The patient's desires for life-prolonging measures must be documented. Patients are asked whether they have made provisions for surrogate decision-making (advance directives) in the event that they become incapacitated, and if they have not, they are encouraged to do so. Important is acclimating patients and their surrogates to discussing goals of care; then, when circumstances necessitate medical judgments and prior documentation is unavailable or irrelevant (which is extremely often), proper decisions can be made.

Remember

If patients recall having surgery but do not remember the procedure or its purpose, surgical records should be obtained if possible.

APPROACH TO AN ELDERLY PATIENT

Evaluation of the elderly typically deviates from the traditional medical evaluation. History-taking and physical examination may need to be performed at various times for older patients, particularly those who are very old or feeble, and physical examination may take two sessions due to patient exhaustion.

The elderly also have unique, frequently more complex health care issues, such as various ailments, which may need the use of multiple prescriptions (commonly referred to as polypharmacy) and increase the possibility that a high-risk drug may be prescribed. Complicated diagnosis may result in delayed, missed, or incorrect diagnoses, leading to improper drug use.

KEYWORD

Social isolation is the lack of social contacts and having few people to interact with regularly.

Early discovery of problems leads to early intervention, which can avoid deterioration and improve life quality, frequently by relatively simple and affordable procedures (eg, lifestyle changes). Some senior patients, particularly those who are frail or chronically unwell, are best examined by a multidisciplinary team employing a thorough geriatric assessment that includes evaluation of function and quality of life.

On average, elderly individuals have six diagnosable conditions, of which the primary care physician is frequently unaware of some. A disease in one organ system can exacerbate the deterioration of another organ system, leading to incapacity, dependence, and death in the absence of intervention. Multiple diseases complicate diagnosis and treatment, and their consequences are exacerbated by social disadvantage (e.g., social isolation) and poverty (as patients outlast their resources and supportive peers) as well as by functional and financial difficulties.

Certain frequent geriatric symptoms (e.g., delirium, dizziness, syncope, falling, mobility issues, weight or appetite loss, and urine incontinence) may be the result of numerous organ system abnormalities, therefore clinicians should pay special attention to these.

KEYWORD

Organ system is a biological system consisting of a group of organs that work together to perform one or more functions.

If a patient has numerous problems, their treatments (e.g. bed rest, surgery, medication) must be well-integrated; treating one disorder without treating adjacent disorders may hasten decline. In addition, rigorous monitoring is required to avoid iatrogenic effects. For instance, with complete bed rest, older individuals can lose between 1% and 3% of muscle mass and strength per day (resulting in sarcopenia), and the effects of bed rest alone can ultimately lead to mortality.

Frequently, prevalent disorders in the elderly are ignored or their diagnosis is delayed. Utilizing the history, physical examination, and simple laboratory testing, clinicians should actively screen senior patients for illnesses that occur only or frequently in the elderly; when discovered early, these problems are frequently more treatable. The clinician's acquaintance with the patient's behavior and history, including mental status, is frequently essential for early identification. Typically, the initial symptoms of a physical disorder are behavioral, mental, or emotional in nature. If clinicians are ignorant of this possibility and attribute these symptoms to dementia, there may be a delay in diagnosis and treatment. In times of pain, cancer, and psychological problems such as delirium, dementia, and Alzheimer's disease, which have been described in previous chapters, health care workers must approach the elderly. A rigorous and comprehensive evaluation of the elderly is essential.

Preliminary Steps (Before you walk into the room)

- Acuity increases with age, so beware of the under-triaged older adult based on:
    - Atypical presentations of common complaints
    - Stoicism or minimization of problem
- Review medical records (if available):
    - Does the patient have a history of dementia, delirium or other cognitive deficit? If so, verify (corroborate) any history

- Is there a pattern of ED(Emergency Department) visits to suggest unmet social needs (e.g. caregiver fatigue; unsafe home environment; poor access to care)
- Are there patterns of injuries to raise suspicion of elder abuse

- Code status and goals of care:
  - information and find out sooner than later

KEYWORD

Psychiatric problem is characterized by a clinically significant disturbance in an individual's cognition, emotional regulation, or behavior.

Recommended Approach and Assessment

Subjective Assessment:

- Older adults may minimize complaints, conditions, and symptoms.
- Over 40% of older adults in ED have a cognitive deficit which may affect history-taking (37% dementia; 5% delirium), corroborate history with family/caregiver/companion whenever feasible to not miss anything.
- Atypical chief complaints are common.
- "Confusion" – Is it dementia, delirium or an intracranial lesion?
  - If they have dementia, how is this episode DIFFERENT FROM BASELINE?
  - A "new" psychiatric problem (e.g. "psychosis" or "mania" or "aggressive behavior" is RARELY a de novo psychiatric problem – think medical (organic) etiology first, then think medications, then think something else OTHER than.
  - Common medical problems can cause change in mutation: UTI; AMI; pain; thyroid dysfunction.

Objective Assessment:

- Mental Status or "Confusion" – Is it dementia, delirium or an intracranial lesion?
  - Not everyone needs a head CT: anyone on anticoagulants MUST get a head CT, EVERYTIME
  - If they have dementia, how is this episode DIFFERENT FROM BASELINE?

- If you suspect undocumented dementia, the Short Blessed Test is a good cognitive function screen for ED use that is most sensitive/specific

- A "new" psychiatric problem (e.g. "psychosis" or "mania" or "aggressive behavior" is RARELY a de novo psychiatric problem – think medical (organic) etiology first, then think medications, then think something else OTHER than psychiatric
- Delirium
  - Richmond Agitation Sedation Scale (RASS) is a quick delirium screen for ED use with very good sensitivity/ specificity; RASS >+1 or <-1 is nearly diagnostic
- Intracranial
  - Older adults, particularly those on anticoagulants, may be at higher risk for delayed bleeds. However, there is NO widely accepted consensus guidelines on screening for delayed bleeds if the initial CT is negative.
  - A compromise strategy may be to screen (e.g. by telephone follow-up for signs/symptoms within 24 hours) to decide the need for repeat head CT within 24 hours of a negative study; if follow-up cannot be guaranteed, admission for observation may be necessary.
- Dizziness
  - 15% of older adults presenting to ED for dizziness have serious etiologies; 4-6% are stroke-related and sensitivity of CT for identifying stroke or intracranial lesion in dizziness is poor (16%), so if CNS etiology is suspected, seek neuro consult or MRI (83% sensitivity).
- Skeletal Injury
  - C-spine injuries may result from seemingly benign trauma/falls.
  - Compression fractures of the vertebral column can result from relatively little trauma.
  - Given high prevalence of osteopenia/osteoporosis, X-ray imaging can have reduced sensitivity, consider CT studies for fractures, especially vertebral fractures
  - Knee pain? May be referred pain from occult hip fracture

Did you get it?

The RASS is one of many sedation scales used in medicine. Other scales include the Ramsay scale, the Sedation-Agitation-Scale, and the COMFORT scale for pediatric patients.

- Cardiopulmonary
  - AMI presents with atypical complaints in older adults (e.g., "indigestion", "dizziness", "tired")
  - The HEART score assigns maximal points to anyone >65y (2 points) but the mean age (+SD) of participants used to derive and validate the HEART score was 61 +15y, thus unclear how valid the score is for the very old.
  - Heart failure (HF): ~70% of patients >65y with HF have normal EF of >50%(18), and BNP (B-type Natriuretic Peptide)underestimates degree of decompensation due to thicker heart (thicker heart, less stretch, smaller rise in BNP); consider BNP difference from last hospital discharge to help determine severity and disposition.
- Abdominal pain
  - Visceral pain is modified in older adults; an exam can underestimate severity.
  - Constipation and urinary retention are common but often overlooked causes of abdominal pain.
  - Risk of ischemic bowel is higher in older adults.
  - Acute abdominal series provides a quick screen for perforation or SBO (Small Bowel Obstruction) and balances the benefit of CT against higher risk of contrast-induced nephropathy in older adults.
- Falls
  - Rule-out medical/surgical or medication-related reasons for the fall; check orthostatic vital signs
  - One mechanical fall in a given year –no unequivocal need for further ED testing unless clinical suspicion
  - Two falls in a given year is a red flag and requires a comprehensive evaluation (in the outpatient setting; ideally by a geriatrician).

KEYWORD

Small bowel obstruction is a partial or complete blockage of the small intestine, which is a part of the digestive system.

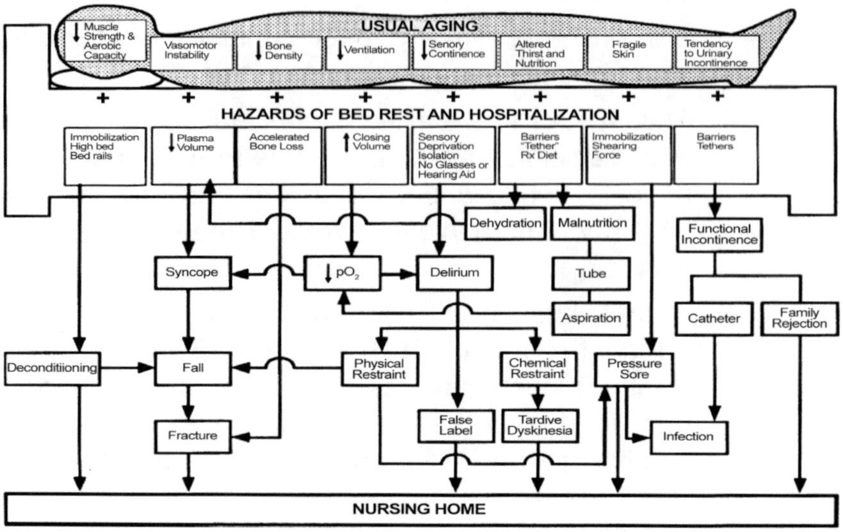

KEYWORD

Benzodiazepines are a class of drugs primarily used for treating anxiety, but they also are effective in treating several other conditions.

Clinical Decision Making and ED Management

- Screening for geriatric syndromes is critical
  - polypharmacy
  - delirium/dementia or fall risk
  - function (independence) and mobility o abuse and neglect
- Geriatric syndromes are individually associated with ED returns and adverse outcomes (e.g. hospitalization, death at 30 days) and must be addressed, not necessarily in the ED if prompt and reliable outpatient follow-up with their PCP(Primary Care Physician) can be arranged
- Beware that screening for adverse outcomes is complicated by the scarcity of reliable instruments (results vary across populations)
- Managing the agitated older adult
  - Try to avoid the use of restraints (if a patient has dementia or is delirious, restraints worsen the situation)
  - Is agitation related to pain? Agitation is often secondary to pain: Start with low dose opioid, and titrate up (start low and go slow) – why? You can reverse it
  - Avoid benzodiazepines with delirium, they can

paradoxically worsen it – UNLESS patient is on chronic benzodiazepines (make sure it's for a good reason), then consider use as it could be benzo withdrawal

- Avoid Haldol – Haldol can lead to fatal reactions in Parkinson's disease and prolonged QT interval; if neither condition is present (once you're sure), then use a LOW dose. AVOID Haldol 5mg in anyone over 55. Use magnesium sulfate to treat long QT interval
- Antipsychotics help manage the behavior but will NOT treat the underlying cause – you still need to evaluate for the medical cause(s) of the agitation

KEYWORD

Antipsychotics are a type of psychiatric medication which are available on prescription to treat psychosis.

- After any diagnostic study with IV contrast, give fluids
  - Older adults are at higher risk of contrast-induced nephropathy; IV saline is recommended.
- IV fluid resuscitation: Unless the patient is in shock, a steady IV infusion is preferred over a rapid bolus, particularly if heart failure present
- Medications
- Do not assume what is listed in the computer accurately reflects the patient's medication regimen
- Always confirm medication regimen with patient, family, or pharmacy/home health if patient/family not able to tell
- Potentially Inappropriate Medications (PIM). Older adults have greater susceptibility to adverse effects of particular medications.
- New symptoms may be due to a medication side effect.
- New medications for common complaints could be a source of adverse outcomes.
- PIMs may be indicated and necessary in specific ED situations (e.g. diphenhydramine for acute allergic reactions) but be cautious regarding duration/course when prescribing for post-discharge use.

Disposition

- Precautionary steps at time of discharge
  - Ability to understand and follow discharge instructions (consider the degree of patient and caregiver health literacy, low vision, cognitive impairment, logistics of clinician follow-up)

- If all work-ups are negative but clinical suspicion persists
    - Pursue rapid (24-48 hours) outpatient follow-up with PCP (if available and if patient logistically can go to PCP)
    - Consider the 48-hour ED return
- CAUTION: Hospitalization worsens function, mobility, and morbidity which in turn leads to ED returns and hospitalization.
    - Hospitalize only if clinically indicated (ideally)
    - If social issues exist – can ED social worker or case manager find a sufficiently safe disposition for the patient and avoid hospitalization?
    - If social needs cannot be met, or if safety is a concern, then admit to the hospital but ensure that inpatient service understands the problem (and document this need for transitions of care)

KEYWORD

Morbidity is when you have a specific illness or condition. Some examples of common morbidities are heart disease, diabetes, and obesity.

Pitfalls

- Look for atypical presentations of common medical conditions.
- Avoid admitting to hospital simply because of their age, as unwarranted hospitalization can be harmful to the patient's subsequent function, mobility, and quality of life.
    - Know your own biases: older adults are a source of stress in EPs; >75% recognize the need to improve the quality of care.
    - 22% of ED admits are potentially avoidable.
    - 50% of ED admits are for non-clinical reasons.
- Address unmet social needs as these are highly responsible for ED returns– ask ED social worker or case manager for help.
- Screen for geriatric syndromes to identify older adults at high risk for adverse events
    - Delirium (abnormal RASS score) predicts increased mortality at 6 months.
    - Dementia is unrecognized in the ED up to 70% of the time.
    - Elder abuse and neglect may have subtle signs/ symptoms.

- Two mechanical falls in a given year indicate an increased risk of adverse events.
- Declines in mobility (e.g. walking speed) are associated with increased hospitalization or mortality.
- Potentially Inappropriate Medications (PIMs)

LEVELS OF GERIATRIC CARE AND ROLES OF THE NURSE

Gerontology (from the Greek geron, "old man" and logia, "study of"; coined by IlyaIlyich Mechnikov in 1903) is the study of the social, cultural, psychological, cognitive, and biological aspects of aging. It is distinguished from geriatrics, which is the branch of medicine that specializes in the treatment of existing disease in older adults. Gerontologists include researchers and practitioners in the fields of biology, nursing, medicine, criminology, dentistry, social work, physical and occupational therapy, psychology, psychiatry, sociology, economics, political science, architecture, geography, pharmacy, public health, housing, and anthropology.

KEYWORD

Gerontology is the study of the social, cultural, psychological, cognitive, and biological aspects of aging.

Gerontology encompasses the following:

- Studying physical, mental, and social changes in people as they age
- Investigating the biological aging process itself including aging's causes, effects and mechanisms (bio gerontology)
- Investigating the social and psycho-social impacts of aging (sociogerontology)
- Investigating the psychological effects on aging (psycho gerontology)
- Investigating the interface of biological aging with aging-related diseases (geroscience)
- Investigating the effects of an aging population on society (demography)
- Exploring the relationship between the aging and their environment (environmental gerontology)
- Applying this knowledge to policies and programs, including the macroscopic (for example, government planning) and microscopic (for example, running a nursing home) perspectives

Due to the multidisciplinary character of gerontology, it overlaps with a variety of subfields and linked subjects, including physiology, anthropology, social work, public health, psychology, and sociology. Geriatric care management (also known as "elder care management", "senior health care management", and "professional care management") is the process of planning and coordinating the care of the elderly and others with physical and/or mental impairments to meet their long-term care needs, improve their quality of life, and preserve their independence for as long as possible. It involves monitoring, providing, and referring several forms of health and social care services to elderly individuals and their families. Geriatric care managers achieve this by combining a working understanding of health and psychology, human development, family dynamics, public and private resources, and funding sources, while advocating for their clients across the continuum of care. For instance, they may provide assistance to the families of older persons and others with chronic requirements, such as those with Alzheimer's disease or another kind of dementia.

Remember

Geriatric care management integrates health care and psychological care with other needed services such as: housing, home care services, nutritional services, assistance with activities of daily living, socialization programs, as well as financial and legal planning (e.g. banking, trusts).

Definitions of Geriatric Care

Care for the elderly, or simply elder care (known in certain areas of the English-speaking world as aged care), is the satisfaction of the specialized demands and requirements of senior persons. This broad phrase includes assisted living, adult day care, long-term care, nursing homes (also known as residential care), hospice care, and home care.

Geriatrics is the medical specialty concerned with the treatment of the aged. It attempts to improve the health of older individuals and to prevent and treat diseases and disabilities.

Gerontological nursing is a subspecialty of nursing that focuses on the care of elderly persons. Gerontological nurses collaborate with older individuals, their families, and their communities to promote healthy aging, optimal functioning, and quality of life. The name gerontological nursing, which superseded geriatric nursing in the 1970s, is viewed as more compatible with the specialty's greater emphasis on health and wellbeing in addition to sickness.

OVERVIEW OF GERIATRIC CARE

Geriatric care management blends health care and mental health care with housing, home care services, dietary services, aid with activities of daily living, socializing programs, and financial and legal planning (e.g. banking, trusts). After a full assessment, a care plan that is suited to the individual's circumstances is established and is regularly monitored and updated as necessary. A thorough assessment of geriatric care can take between 2 and 5 hours, which is split down into 2 or 3 patient/family assessment visits. The comprehensive assessment is actually a collection of smaller individual examinations, the first of which is a primary intake assessment that contains demographic information, a health history, a social history, and a legal/financial history. A medication profile assessment and an assessment of ADLs (Activities of Daily Living) and IADLs (Instruments of Activities of Daily Living) follow (Instrumental Activities of Daily Living). In addition, additional assessments may include a falls risk assessment, a home safety assessment, a nutritional assessment, a depression assessment, a pain assessment, the Mini Mental State Exam (MMSE), the MiniCog Clock Drawing Exam (Cognitive Assessment), a balance assessment, and a gait assessment (ability to walk). If the comprehensive geriatric care management assessment is being conducted by a Registered Health Care Professional, a physical assessment such as recording vital signs such as temperature, pulse, respirations, blood pressure, oxygen saturation, and occasionally FBS or RBS (Fasting or Random Blood Sugar) checks for diabetics may be included. In addition, physical evaluations in areas including cardiopulmonary, gastrointestinal, musculoskeletal, genitourinary, eyes/ears/nose/throat, integumentary (skin), lower extremities inspection, a modified neuro assessment, and a medication compliance assessment.

KEYWORD

Nutritional assessment allows healthcare providers to systematically assess the overall nutritional status of patients, diagnose malnutrition, identify underlying pathologies that lead to malnutrition, and plan necessary interventions.

Due to their propensity for various illnesses and possible social or functional issues, older persons consume a disproportionately significant amount of health care resources. In the US, people ≥ 65 account for:

- > 40% of acute hospital bed days.
- > 30% of prescription and OTC drug purchases.
- $329 billion or almost 44% of the national health budget.
- > 75% of the federal health budget.

The elderly are likely to see multiple health care professionals and migrate between health care settings. Providing consistent, integrated treatment across specialized care settings, also referred to as continuity of care, is crucial for senior people. Communication among primary care physicians, specialists, other health care practitioners, patients, and their families is crucial for ensuring that patients receive appropriate care in all settings, particularly when patients are transferred between settings. The use of electronic medical records may facilitate communication.

Health Care Settings for Providing Geriatric Care

Geriatric care may be delivered in the following settings:

- Physician's office: Routine diagnosis and management of acute and chronic disorders, health promotion and disease prevention, and pre-surgical or post-surgical evaluation are the most frequent reasons for visits.
- Patient's home: Home care is utilized most frequently following hospital release; however, hospitalization is not a must. In addition, a small but growing number of health care professionals provide acute and chronic care, as well as end-of-life care, in the patient's home.
- Long-term care facilities include assisted living communities, board-and-care homes, nursing homes, and life-care communities. Whether a patient requires care in a long-term care facility depends in part on the patient's desires and needs, as well as the family's capacity to meet those needs.
- Day care facilities: These facilities provide medical, rehabilitative, cognitive, and social services several hours a day for several days a week.
- Only very ill elderly persons should be hospitalized in hospitals. Due to confinement, immobility, diagnostic tests, and therapies, hospitalization itself offers hazards to senior individuals.
- Hospices provide care for the terminally ill. The objective is to reduce symptoms and keep individuals comfortable, as opposed to curing the condition. Hospice care might be administered in the patient's residence, a nursing home, or an inpatient institution.
- Senior Communities: Senior living is meant for independent seniors who do not require assistance with ADLs. Senior communities are typically age-restricted neighborhoods or towns. There are a range of social clubs, including golf, arts and crafts, and card games, that are created for active seniors. While some senior communities provide additional levels of care, the majority are not equipped to assist those with ADLs. Some senior living facilities compel residents to relocate if they require this degree of care.
- Continuing Care: Communities that provide continuing care are often known as "step care" or "progressive"

KEYWORD

Immobility mean the condition of not being able to move, like that poor mouse stuck in a glue trap whose immobility will lead to its starvation.

care facilities. They provide a variety of possibilities, from independent living to special care. Typically, residents are admitted when they live independently. As their demands increase, slots in the lower level of care are guaranteed. Typically, an admission fee is required, making this alternative rather costly.

- Assisted Living: Assisted living provides senior citizens with a place to live outside of their own home, where they can receive basic assistance in one or more of the following areas: housekeeping, meal preparation, 24/7 monitoring, shower assistance, toileting, medication assistance or reminders, transportation, eating, dressing, activities, or socialization. Your loved one will typically have their own apartment in assisted living, unless you or your loved one consent to room sharing. Most apartments provide a separate bathroom for the sake of privacy and dignity. Most apartments will include a kitchenette with a sink, microwave, refrigerator, and cabinet space. Each apartment will likely have its own climate control system. Common amenities will include a TV room, exercise room, dining room, library, and communal sitting places. People who require assistance with complicated ADLs on a daily basis reside in assisted living facilities. Included among the ADLs are eating, bathing, dressing, and hygiene. Complex ADLs involve shopping, cooking, and managing money. The objective of assisted living is to bridge the gap between independent living and long-term care. The majority of assisted living facilities provide a dining area designed to resemble a restaurant as well as a selection of activities. Most assisted living facilities are not authorized to deliver intravenous fluids, necessitating that patients who require IVs shift temporarily to a skilled nursing facility.
- Board and Care: Board and care is comparable to assisted living in terms of care, although some group homes serve seniors with a lesser level of functionality than those in assisted living. This is typically a single-family home that has been converted into housing for the elderly and disabled. In addition to a 24-hour staff member, monthly rent typically includes lodging, three meals per day, laundry services, and some transportation. While people with major medical concerns will be expected to migrate to a more suitable facility, basic medical treatment will be provided.
- Skilled Nursing: Skilled nursing (sometimes referred to as

KEYWORD

Climate control system is a complex system that requires routine maintenance for increased seasonal performance and operation.

SNF or "sniff") is the first licensed level of care in which nurses administer medical therapy. In fact, nurses are required by law to be on duty and the nurse-to-patient ratio is strictly regulated. As the name suggests, this type of facility provides comprehensive nursing care to its inhabitants. Admission must be initiated by a person's physician, who recommends that a patient enter either 'rehab care' or a 'special care' facility.

- *Rehab care*: Located in hospitals or nursing homes, rehab care programs are sometimes called "Level 1" or transitional care. They provide intensive medical care for patients who are expected to regain functional capacity and return home in a relatively short time.
- *Special care*: There are two types of special care facilities: those involved with unique medical issues (sometimes called "Level 2" care), and those which manage behavioral problems that may arise from dementia.

KEYWORD

Intravenous antibiotics are antibiotics that are administered directly into a vein so that they can enter the bloodstream immediately and bypass the absorption in the gut.

Many patients are admitted to skilled nursing facilities to treat an acute ailment, such as the rehabilitation of a fractured hip or the treatment of an infection with intravenous antibiotics. Many skilled nursing institutions have a percentage of long-term care patients as residents. These individuals require the therapeutic capabilities of an SNF but require this level of care permanently because of their illness. Long-term care includes nursing supervision, but is of a custodial type, with a focus on maintenance rather than treatment. Here, it is not anticipated that the patient's condition would improve, hence the focus of nursing care is on maintaining the patient's health and safety.

Principles of Geriatric Care

- Clinical judgment should be used to determine which level of care would be most appropriate based on the criteria below.
- Although a lower level of care will typically necessitate a lower nurse-to-patient ratio or reduced critical care support, this may not always be the case, and the goal should be to provide flexible staff resources to meet the patient's needs. The degree of care allocated to a patient will influence staffing requirements but will not determine them.
- Patients' level of care is not determined by their location.

- Patients who have resuscitation orders written or who are receiving palliative care may also fulfill the criteria listed below. It may be necessary to modify the actual amount of intensive care provided to these individuals while simultaneously strengthening their palliative care.

KEYWORD

Personal care services are hands-on services that assist a person with critical day-to-day activities that they are unable to perform on their own.

Services of Geriatric Care

Home Health

- Services must be ordered by a doctor.
- Services may include nurse, home health aide, therapies (ot, speech, pt).
- Services are provided in the patient's place of residence.
- Services may include assistance with all or some of ADLs.
- Services may be long or short term.
- Patient may be dependent, semi-independent, and have acute or chronic health status.
- Services are on an intermittent basis, not 24 hours a day.
- Patient participates in a plan of care developed by a RN.
- Personal care services (ADLs) provided according to R432-700-30, which include dressing, eating, grooming, bathing, toileting, ambulation, transferring, and self-administration of medications.

Assisted Living Facility Type I

- Resident lives in a licensed facility that provides safe and clean-living accommodations and three meals a day.
- Resident may require minimal assistance with ADLs, including significant assistance with up to two ADLs.
- Resident must be able to evacuate the facility under his own power (be mobile).
- Resident must have stable health and free from any communicable disease.
- Resident may receive assistance with medications or have medications administered by a nurse.
- Resident may receive home health services through an individual contract with a home health agency.
- Resident receives 24-hour general monitoring, 7 days a week.

- Resident may receive general nursing care according to facility policy.
- Resident participates in developing a service plan.

Assisted Living Facility Type II

- Resident lives in a licensed facility, permits aging in place.
- Resident may receive full assistance with ADLs.
- Resident may be semi-independent and may require the assistance of one person for transfers or to evacuate the facility.
- Resident may receive assistance with medication or have medications administered by a nurse.
- Resident receives general nursing care from facility staff.
- Resident must be free of communicable diseases that could be transmitted to others through the normal course of activities.
- Resident receives 24-hour individualized personal and health-related services, 7 days a week.
- Resident may receive home health services through individual contract with a home health agency.
- Resident participates in developing a service plan.

Did you get it?

Health services refer to the range of activities, facilities, and resources provided to individuals and communities to promote, maintain, and improve their health and well-being.

Small Health Care Facility - Type n - (Limited to Three Persons)

- Resident lives in a licensed home occupied by the owner or operator.
- Resident receives supervised nursing care on a daily basis from a written plan of care.
- Resident receives assistance with medications or receives medication administration by a nurse.
- Resident must be free of communicable diseases and does not require 24-hour nursing care or inpatient.

Hospital Care

- Resident may be dependent.
- Resident may receive total assist with ADLs.
- Resident receives 24 hour direct care staff for monitoring and assistance.
- Resident may receive rehabilitative services through

individual contract with a home health agency.

Intermediate Care Facilities/Nursing Facilities

Resident lives in a licensed facility that provides 24-hour inpatient care to residents who need licensednursing supervision and supportive care, but do not require continuous nursing care.

- Resident may be semi-independent or dependent.
- Resident may receive full assistance with ADLs.
- Resident may receive full assistance with transfers.
- Resident receives medications from a nurse following a doctor's order.
- Resident may receive outpatient rehab services.
- Facility provides licensed nursing coverage 8 hours a day for facilities with less than 35 beds and 16 hours for facilities with 35 or more beds. Facilities have run as consultant.
- Resident receives periodic assessments by a licensed practitioner.

KEYWORD

Periodic assessment is an opportunity for learners to draw on a range of learning that has taken place over an extended period of time.

Skilled Nursing Facility

- Resident lives in a licensed facility that provides 24-hour licensed nursing services, eight hours of which is RN coverage.
- Resident may be dependent and require total assistance with ADLs.
- Resident receives medications from a nurse according to a licensed practitioner's order.
- Resident receives required rehab services from the facility.

Hospital

- Patient is admitted to a licensed facility for a short term for a condition that requires treatment.
- Patient receives 24-hour RN care.
- Patient may receive rehab services either inpatient or outpatient.
- Patient may be dependent and require full assistance with ADLs.

- Patient receives medications from an RN according to the licensed practitioner's orders.

Hospice

- The hospice program is a health care agency or facility that offers palliative and supportive services providing physical, psychological, social and spiritual care for dying persons and their families.
- Patient may receive services in their place of residence or an inpatient setting.
- Family and patient participates in a plan of care developed by an interdisciplinary team which includes at least the patient and the patient's family or primary care giver, nurse, social worker, volunteer, and clergy.
- Services must be ordered by a physician.
- Services may include nurse, social worker, clergy, volunteer, physical therapy, occupational therapy, speech therapy, nutritional therapy, and home health aides.

KEYWORD

Social worker is a trained professional who works with all types of vulnerable people, groups, and communities to help them learn to live better lives.

Geriatric Interdisciplinary Team

Geriatric multidisciplinary teams are composed of practitioners from many disciplines who provide coordinated, integrated care in accordance with collaboratively determined objectives and shared resources and responsibilities. Not all elderly people require a structured interdisciplinary geriatric team. However, when patients have complex medical, psychological, and social needs, such teams are more effective than practitioners working alone in assessing patient needs and developing an appropriate care plan. If interdisciplinary care is not available, a geriatrician or a primary care physician with experience and an interest in geriatric medicine can provide care.

Interdisciplinary teams have the following objectives:

- That patients move safely and readily from one care environment to another and from one practitioner to another.
- That the best qualified practitioner treats each concern.
- That care is not duplicated.

To design, monitor, or amend the care plan, interprofessional teams must communicate routinely and openly. Core team members must organize the care plan collaboratively, with trust and appreciation for the contributions of others (e.g., by delegating, sharing accountability, jointly implementing it). It is possible for team members to work at the same location, making communication informal and quick.

A team normally consists of physicians, nurses, pharmacists, social workers, and occasionally a dietitian, physical and occupational therapists, an ethicist, or a physician specializing in hospice care. Members of the team must have understanding of geriatric medicine, familiarity with the patient, commitment to the team process, and effective communication skills.

KEYWORD

Information technology (IT) is the use of any computers, storage, networking and other physical devices, infrastructure and processes to create, process, store, secure and exchange all forms of electronic data.

Teams need a formal framework to function efficiently. Teams should establish timelines for achieving their objectives, hold regular meetings (to review team structure, methodology, and communication), and check their progress continually (using quality improvement measures). In general, team leadership should rotate based on the patient's needs; the primary provider of care should report on the patient's development. If the primary issue is the patient's medical condition, for instance, a physician leads the meeting and introduces the patient and family to the team. The physician identifies the patient's medical issues, informs the team (including alternative diagnoses), and explains how these conditions affect care. The input of the team is incorporated into medical orders. The physician is responsible for writing medical orders based on team decisions and discusses team decisions with the patient, family, and care givers.

A virtual team can be utilized if a formally established interdisciplinary team is unavailable or impractical. Typically, the primary care physician leads these teams, but an advanced practice nurse, a care coordinator, or a case manager can form and manage them. The virtual team utilizes information technology (such as handheld devices, email, video conferencing, and teleconferencing) to interact and work with team members in the community or within the health care system.

Patient and Caregiver Participation

Practitioner team members must treat patients and caregivers as active members of the team in the following ways:

- Patients and caregivers should be included in team meetings when appropriate.

- Patients should be asked to help the team set goals (e.g., advance directives, end-of-life care).
- Patients and caregivers should be included in discussions of drug treatment, rehabilitation, dietary plans, and other therapies.
- Patients should be asked what their ideas and preferences are; thus, if patients will not take a particular drug or change certain dietary habits, care can be modified accordingly.

KEYWORD

Health care is the improvement of health via the prevention, diagnosis, treatment, amelioration or cure of disease, illness, injury, and other physical and mental impairments in people.

Patients and practitioners must communicate honestly to prevent patients from suppressing an opinion and agreeing to every suggestion. Patients with cognitive impairments should be included in decision-making, provided that practitioners communicate at a level that patients can comprehend. The capacity to make decisions regarding health care is decision-specific; people who are incapable of making sophisticated judgments may nevertheless be competent to make decisions on less complex issues.

Based on the patient's behaviors and lifestyle, caregivers, including family members, might aid by recognizing realistic and unrealistic expectations. Caregivers should also indicate the type of assistance they can offer.

Typically, geriatric care managers have a background in nursing, social work, gerontology, or other health service fields. It is assumed that they have in-depth knowledge of the pricing, quality, and availability of services in their communities. In certain nations and jurisdictions, certification may be obtained from various professional groups, such as the National Association of Professional Geriatric Care Managers in the United States.

Professional care managers help individuals, families and other caregivers adjust and cope with the challenges of aging or disability by:

- Conducting care-planning assessments to identify needs, problems and eligibility for assistance.
- Screening, arranging, and monitoring in-home help and other services.
- Reviewing financial, legal, or medical issues.
- Offering referrals to specialists to avoid future problems and to conserve assets.
- Providing crisis intervention.

- Acting as a liaison to families at a distance.
- Making sure things are going well and alerting families of problems.
- Assisting with moving their clients to or from a retirement complex, assisted living facility, rehabilitation facility or nursing home.
- Providing client and family education and advocacy.
- Offering counseling and support.

Depending on the country and health care institution, geriatric care managers' professional costs may be billed privately on a fee-for-service basis. They are not covered by Medicaid, Medicare, or the majority of commercial health insurance policies in the United States. Depending on the individual's case history, clients may be able to submit bills for some services to their long-term care insurance.

KEYWORD

Self-esteem is how we value and perceive ourselves. It's based on our opinions and beliefs about ourselves, which can feel difficult to change.

Role of a Nurse in Geriatric Care

Maintaining the patient's physical safety, reducing anxiety and agitation, improving communication, promoting independence in self-care activities, meeting the patient's needs for socialization, self-esteem, and intimacy, ensuring adequate nutrition, managing sleep pattern disturbances, and providing support and education to family caregivers are the goals of nursing interventions. When the nurse can provide such assistance, older persons are able to maintain greater levels of perceived and actual health, according to research.

As the patient's cognitive ability drops, the nurse creates a calm, predictable atmosphere that enables the individual to interpret his or her surroundings and activities. Environmental stimuli are restricted, and a regimen is adhered to. A calm, pleasant tone of voice, clear and simple explanations, and the use of memory aids and cues help to reduce confusion and disorientation and instill a sense of confidence in the patient. Clocks and calendars prominently displayed may facilitate orientation to time. If a patient has trouble locating his or her room, color-coding the door may be of assistance. Active participation may prolong the patient's cognitive, functional, and social interaction skills. Physical activity and communication have also been shown to retard cognitive deterioration.

Promoting Physical Safety

A safe environment permits the patient to move as freely as possible and relieves the patient's family of constant safety concerns. All obvious risks are eliminated to prevent falls and other injuries. Nightlights are advantageous. The patient's medication and food consumption is tracked. Smoking is only permitted under supervision. A risk-free environment affords the patient the greatest degree of independence and autonomy. Due to a short attention span and amnesia, a patient's wandering behavior can typically be controlled through gentle persuasion or distraction. Because restraints have the potential to promote agitation, they are avoided. The doors leading outside must be secured. To protect the patient, all activities must be supervised outside the home, and he or she must wear an identity bracelet or necklace in case he or she becomes separated from the caregiver.

KEYWORD

Cognitive impairment is when a person has trouble remembering, learning new things, concentrating, or making decisions that affect their everyday life.

Reducing Anxiety and Agitation

Despite severe cognitive impairments, the patient will occasionally be aware of his or her fast deteriorating abilities. The patient requires ongoing emotional care that promotes a good self-image. When skill loss occurs, goals are modified to accommodate the patient's declining ability. The surroundings should be uncluttered, comfortable, and quiet. The angry, combative mood known as a catastrophic reaction can be triggered by excitement and confusion, which can be unsettling (over-reaction to excessive stimulation). During such a reaction, the patient responds with screams, tears, or hostility (physically or verbally). This may be the only way the patient can show an inability to cope with the surrounding environment. When this occurs, it is essential to remain calm and composed. Listening to music, petting, rocking, or distracting the patient may calm him or her. The patient frequently forgets what sparked the emotion. Additionally, structuring tasks is beneficial. The ability to anticipate the patient's responses to specific stimuli enables caregivers to avoid similar circumstances.

Late-stage dementia patients often remain in nursing facilities and receive the majority of their care from nursing assistants. To reduce patient agitation, dementia education for caregivers is essential and is given very well by advanced practice nurse specialists.

Improving Communication

To facilitate the patient's comprehension of communications, the nurse should maintain a calm demeanor and minimize background noise. Because patients typically forget the meaning of words or have trouble organizing and articulating their thoughts, it is crucial that messages be conveyed using clear, simple language. In the beginning, lists and straightforward written directions may be useful. In the later stages, the patient may be able to communicate by pointing to objects or using nonverbal language. Generally, tactile inputs such as hugs and hand pats are regarded as indications of care, concern, and safety.

KEYWORD

Nonverbal language refers to the use of gestures, facial expressions, body language, posture, eye contact, and other nonverbal cues to convey meaning and express emotions without the use of words.

Because interaction with friends and family can be reassuring, visits, letters, and phone conversations are encouraged to meet socialization and intimacy needs. Visits should be quick and stress-free; limiting the number of guests to one or two at a time helps prevent overstimulation. Recreation is essential, and individuals are encouraged to engage in simple activities. Realistic objectives are appropriate for activities that offer satisfaction. Hobbies and activities such as walking, exercising, and interacting with others can enhance life quality. A pet's nonjudgmental friendliness can induce calm and bring fulfillment. Plant and animal care can be gratifying and a source of energy.

The elderly and their partners can engage in sexual activity. They should be encouraged to discuss any sexual problems. Simple displays of affection, such as holding and touching, are frequently profound.

Mealtime can be a joyful social occasion or a time of sorrow and misery; therefore, it should be kept simple, quiet, and confrontation-free. People want foods that are both attractive and delicious. To prevent fiddling with food, serve each dish separately. Cut food into little pieces to prevent choking. If liquids are turned to gelatin, they may be simpler to swallow. To prevent burns, hot foods and beverages are served warm.

Promoting Balanced Activity and Rest

Many people complain of sleep difficulties and potentially improper wandering behaviors. These behaviors are more likely to occur when bodily or psychological demands are unmet. Caregivers must detect the requirements of patients showing these behaviors, as their health may deteriorate further if they are not addressed.

During the day, physical activity can be encouraged while daytime sleep for extended periods is discouraged.

Did you Know?

A geriatric nursing specialty group was formed by the American Nurses Association in 1966, with the name changed to the Gerontological Nursing Division in 1976.

Supporting Home and Community Based Care

The emotional burden on the families of elderly are enormous. Typically, the physical health is stable and mental decline is gradual. Family members may confront challenging decisions. The older peoples' anger and agitation are frequently misconstrued by their families. Abuse and neglect of older individuals must be avoided, and they must be continually monitored for minor and significant disorders that require rapid medical attention.

REVIEW QUESTIONS

1. Describe the scope and concept of gerontological nursing.
2. Explain how the attitude of people influences the care of the elderly.
3. Elaborate on the history of gerontological nursing.
4. Define gerontological nursing. Explain in detail the various principles of gerontological nursing.
5. Define geriatric assessment. Explain in detail the various approaches for assessment of the elderly.

MULTIPLE CHOICE QUESTIONS

1. A 66-year-old recently widowed patient with limited income is planning to move into the home of her daughter and son-in-law and their two adolescent children in order to share expenses, and she is concerned about the transition and a lack of independence. The best advice is for the patient to

a. accept the changes in her life.

b. apply for low-cost housing elsewhere.

c. set the ground rules for living together.

d. have a frank discussion with the family.

2. If a patient is severely dehydrated, what effect will this have on the complete blood count (CBC)?

a. Increased hemoglobin and hematocrit, decreased blood volume, and stable red blood cell (RBC) count.

b. Decreased hemoglobin and hematocrit, decreased blood volume, and increased RBC count.

c. Decreased hemoglobin and hematocrit, decreased blood volume, and decreased RBC count.

d. Stable hemoglobin and hematocrit decreased blood volume and stable RBC count.

3. The gerontological nurse is working in a mobile clinic to provide care to a homeless population. Among the older adults in this population, the health problems that the gerontological nurse most expects to find include:

a. psychiatric/substance abuse disorders.

b. neurological disorders.

c. digestive disorders.

d. traumatic injuries.

4. **The gerontological nurse is monitoring signs of suspected abuse in an 89-year-old patient who was admitted from home. When planning for the patient's discharge, the nurse's first action is to:**
   a. delay discharge by informing the provider of the suspected abuse.
   b. enlist the help of family members with transitioning the patient home.
   c. notify Adult Protective Services of the patient's discharge.
   d. restrict the family members' access to the patient prior to discharge.
5. **A resident in a nursing home requests a new room because he or she does not like the view from the current room. While the resident is away from the home on a provider visit, the staff moves the resident's belongings to another room with a better view. The resident and the resident's family later file a formal complaint regarding the move. Which statement gives the best justification for the resident's complaint?**
   a. The change was made without a provider's order.
   b. The resident was not included in the decision-making.
   c. The resident's belongings were moved without his or her assistance.
   d. The resident's family was not included in the decision making.

Answers to Multiple Choice Questions

1. (d) 2. (a) 3. (a) 4. (c) 5. (b)

REFERENCES

1. Suzanne C. Smeltzer (2004), textbook of medical surgical nursing, 12th edition, Lippincott William and Wilkins publishers, p185-210.
2. Lewis (2010), Textbook of medical surgical nursing, 9th edition, Elsevier publishers, p120-138
3. Gerentological Nursing- Competencies of care by Kristen L. Mauk Jones & Bartlett Publishers, 2010

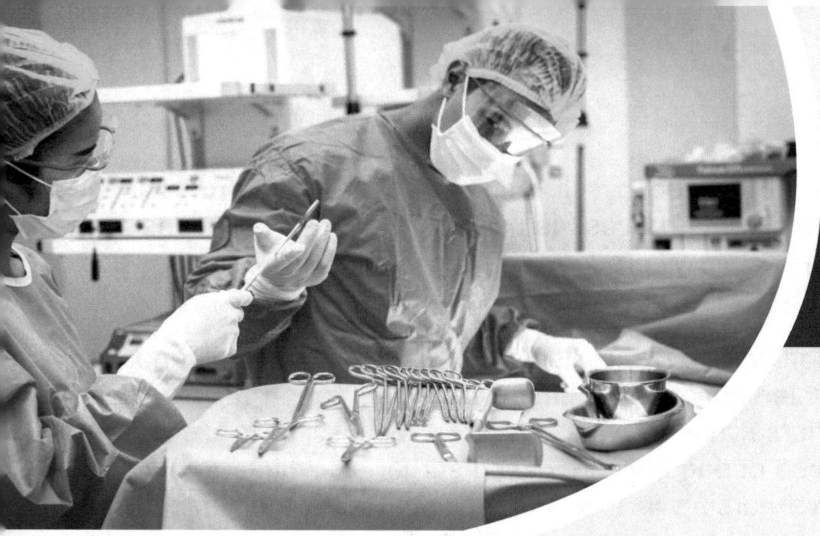

CHAPTER 7

PERIOPERATIVE NURSING

"Nurses are there when the last breath is taken, and nurses are there when the first breath is taken. Although it is more enjoyable to celebrate the birth, it is just as important to comfort in death."

—Christine Belle

INTRODUCTION

Numerous diseases and injuries require surgical or procedural intervention for therapy. During surgery, the skills and abilities of multiple healthcare professionals are merged for the patient's benefit. Surgery may be performed for a variety of reasons, including: to cure or minimize disease; to diagnose the specific presence of a disease or condition; to reconstruct or eliminate a defect; to enhance form and function; to prescribe appropriate postoperative treatment and prognosis; to palliate, or offer comfort, when cure is not possible; to follow up or monitor an incurable disease process; and to offer a preventative option when disease is inevitable, such as an elective, prophylactic procedure. Any physical part or system may be the subject of planned or unplanned, elective/optional or essential, major or small surgery. Surgery is a stressful event that necessitates physical and psychological adjustments for the patient and his or her family. Whether the operation is performed as an outpatient or in the hospital, the patient's recuperation following surgery requires skilled and competent nursing care.

Perioperative nursing refers to the care offered to the patient before, during, and after surgery. The perioperative continuum consists of the patient's preoperative, intraoperative, and postoperative stages. This word is utilized by all members of the interprofessional team, including the nursing staff. The nursing process is used to conduct evaluations and give interventions to improve health recovery, prevent additional injury or disease, and facilitate adaptation to changes in physical structure and function.

The type of scheduled operation impacts the desired results, nursing diagnoses, nursing assessments, and nursing interventions. For instance, when caring for a patient undergoing same-day surgery, the nurse may provide care from admission to discharge. Typically, the responsibility of the nurse during hospital-based surgery is limited to a single phase. The objective of perioperative nursing is to encourage and help the patient and family in achieving a level of health equal to or greater than that which existed previous to the surgery.

Learning Objectives

After completing the chapter, you will be able to accomplish the following:

- Define the surgical experience
- Explain the nursing process for preoperative care
- Teaching about surgical events and sensations

Key-Terms

- Postoperative phase
- Nurse interventions
- General anesthesia
- Regional anesthesia
- Caudal anesthesia
- Anxiety
- Hyperkalemia

THE SURGICAL EXPERIENCE

Regardless of the required surgical or interventional technique or the setting in which it is performed, all patients must undergo particular phases, get anesthetic and monitoring support, and provide informed consent for surgery.

Phases of the Perioperative Period

During the perioperative period, the patient undergoes surgery through various unique phases. The three phases of perioperative patient care are as follows:

- The preoperative phase, which begins when both the patient and surgeon agree that surgery is necessary and will occur. It concludes with the transport of the patient to the operating room (OR) or procedure bed.
- The intraoperative phase, beginning when the patient is transferred to the OR bed, also called a table, until transfer to the postoperative recovery area.
- The postoperative phase, lasting from admission to the recovery area to complete recovery from surgery and the last follow-up physician visit.

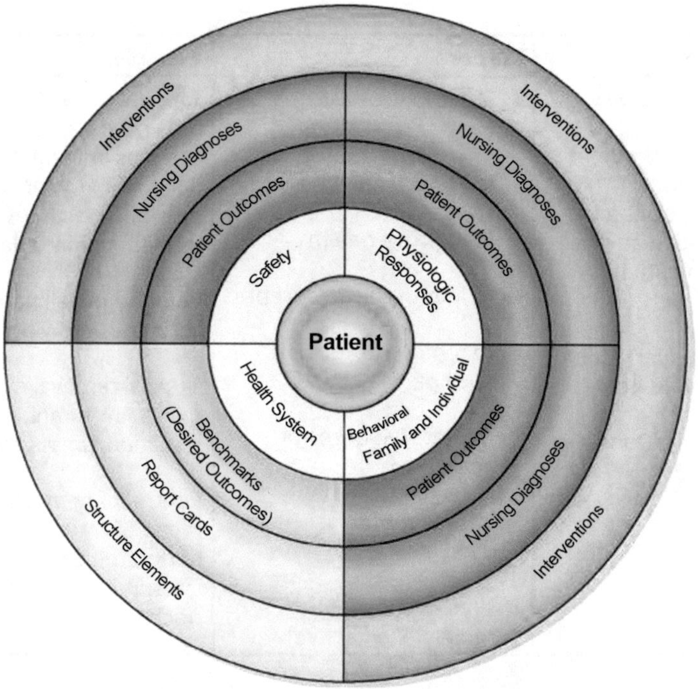

Figure 7.1. Association of perioperative Registered Nurses Perioperative Patient-Focused Model.

The postoperative phase can be further subdivided into phases I (providing patient care from a totally anesthetized state to one requiring less acute nursing interventions), II (preparing the patient for self or family care or care in a phase III extended care environment), and III (providing ongoing care for patients requiring extended observation or intervention after transfer or discharge from phase I or II).

KEYWORD

Psychosocial need include recognition and management of depression, anxiety, fear, developmental problems, disability, pain, and limitations in daily living.

With an increasing tendency toward same-day or short-stay surgical procedures, the nurse interventions in each phase of perioperative nursing care may change slightly, but are essentially identical. Throughout each phase, the nursing process is utilized to address the patient's physical and psychosocial needs and support his or her return to health.

Surgical Procedure Classification

Surgical procedures are often categorized based on urgency, risk, and purpose. The classifications and their respective functions and examples are listed in Table 7.1. Regardless of the established degree of risk, any surgical treatment causes physical and psychological stress on the patient and is rarely regarded as small.

Table 7.1: Classification of surgical procedures

Classification	Purpose	Examples
Based on Urgency Elective: Delay of surgery has no ill effects; can be scheduled in advance based on patient's choice. Urgent: Usually done within 24-48 hours Emergency: Done immediately	• To remove or repair a body part • To restore function • To improve health • To improve self-concept • To remove or repair a body part • To preserve or restore health • To prevent further tissue damage To preserve life (plus purposes listed above)	Tonsillectomy, hernia repair, cataract extraction and lens implantation, hemorrhoidectomy, hip prosthesis, scar revision, facelift, mammoplasty Removal of gallbladder, coronary artery bypass, surgical removal of a malignant tumor, colon resection, amputation Control of hemorrhage; repair of trauma, perforated ulcer, intestinal obstruction; tracheostomy

Based on Degree of Risk Major: May be elective, urgent, or emergency Minor: Primarily elective	• To preserve life • To remove or repair a body part • To restore function • To improve or maintain health • To remove skin lesions To correct deformities	Carotid endarterectomy, cholecystectomy, nephrectomy, colostomy, hysterectomy, radical mastectomy, amputation, trauma repair Teeth extraction, removal of warts, skin biopsy, dilation and curettage, laparoscopy, cataract extraction, arthroscopy
Based on Purpose Diagnostic Ablative Palliative Reconstructive Transplantation Constructive	• To make or confirm a diagnosis • To remove a diseased body part • To relieve or reduce intensity of an illness; is not curative • To restore function to traumatized or malfunctioning tissue • To improve self-concept • To replace organs or structures that are diseased or malfunctioning • To restore function in congenital anomalies	Breast biopsy, laparoscopy, bronchoscopy, exploratory laparotomy Appendectomy, subtotal thyroidectomy, partial gastrectomy, colon resection, amputation Colostomy, nerve root resection, debridement of necrotic tissue, balloon angioplasties, arthroscopy Scar revision, plastic surgery, skin graft, internal fixation of a fracture, breast reconstruction Kidney, liver, cornea, heart, joints Cleft palate repair, closure of atrial-septal defect

Remember

Emergency surgery is designed to deal quickly with problems that can be life-threatening. It involves resuscitation and stabilization of the patient by a patient management team, preparing the patient for surgery, and post-operative and recovery procedures.

Surgery Based on Urgency

Surgery is also categorized into broad categories that cross specialty areas:

- Elective surgery is a procedure that is preplanned and based on the patient's choice and availability of scheduling for the patient, surgeon, and facility. This is a nonurgent procedure that does not have to be done immediately.
- Emergency surgery must be done immediately to preserve life, a body part, or function.

- Urgent surgery must be done within a reasonably short time frame to preserve health, but is not an emergency.
- Optional surgery is not critical to survival or function.

Surgery Based on Degree of Risk

Surgery is categorized as minor or major according to the patient's risk level. Perioperative Nursing is usually always developed in settings such as a physician's office, outpatient clinic, or same-day, outpatient surgical facility. This rating indicates that the surgical operation is often quick, low-risk, and results in few problems. In contrast, major surgery may necessitate hospitalization and specialist care, is typically lengthy, involves major organs or life-threatening conditions, and carries a higher risk of postoperative problems. Due to the tremendous growth of surgical knowledge and technology, however, the major and minor classifications no longer adequately describe the real procedures. Laser technology and minimally invasive techniques involving very small incisions have made major surgery less stressful, necessitating shorter hospitalizations. Even though they are categorized as major, many surgical operations can now be performed on an outpatient (same-day) basis or during a 23-hour hospital stay. Major treatments can be performed with minimal sedation and in a short amount of time, allowing the patient to return home the same day with minimal pain and a speedy return to normal life. New minimally invasive surgical procedures continue to evolve, which will likely continue to influence perioperative care.

Did you Know?

Surgical nursing salaries start just under $70,000 for staff nurses in the United States and can increase to well over $100,000 for OR nurses working in advanced clinical and administrative positions.

Surgery Based on Purpose

Some terms used to classify surgical procedures based on purpose include diagnostic, curative, preventative, ablative, palliative, reconstructive, transplantation, and constructive (see Table 7.1).

Anesthesia

Anesthesia is a strategy and technique for making potentially unpleasant procedures safe and manageable. To inhibit nerve conduction, anesthetic drugs can be delivered systemically, to the entire body, or selectively. General anesthesia, also known as systemic anesthesia, is a combination of unconsciousness, analgesia (pain reduction), relaxation, and lack of reflexes (temporary paralysis). Regional anesthesia, in contrast, does not induce narcosis or drowsiness, but rather analgesia and loss of reflexes. Anesthesiologists (medical doctors) or certified registered nurse anesthetists (CRNA) give anesthetics while monitoring the patient's physiologic reaction and preserving homeostasis during the procedure and recovery. Nurse anesthesia is a subspecialty of advanced nursing. Physicians and nurses who deliver anesthesia conduct preoperative physical examinations, provide preoperative education, administer anesthesia during the surgical operation, and monitor the patient's recovery from the anesthetic.

KEYWORD

Anesthesia is a state of controlled, temporary loss of sensation or awareness that is induced for medical or veterinary purposes.

General Anesthesia

General anesthesia involves the inhalation or intravenous (IV) administration of medications that depress the central nervous system. Typically, general anesthesia is a combination of intravenous and inhalational anesthetics. Loss of consciousness, analgesia, relaxed skeletal muscles, and suppressed reflexes are the desired effects of general anesthesia. After consultation with the patient, the anesthesiologist determines the route and kind of anesthetic administered. These decisions are influenced by a variety of circumstances, including the type and duration of surgery, as well as the patient's physical and mental health. Inhalation anesthesia is frequently utilized due to its quick induction, elimination, and reversal of effects.

Induction, maintenance, and emergence are the three phases of general anesthesia. Induction commences with the administration of the anesthetic agent and continues until the patient is prepared for incision. Maintenance will continue from this point until the procedure's conclusion. Emergence begins when the patient begins to emerge from the altered condition created by anesthesia and often concludes when the patient is ready to leave the operating room; the duration is dependent on the level and duration of anesthesia (Rothrock, 2007). New anesthetic drugs allow patients to "awaken" and emerge from anesthesia in a fraction of the time necessary in the past. As the prevalence of these agents increases, patients typically bypass the PACU. This will allow doctors to perform more surgical procedures in their clinics.

General anesthesia is helpful because it can be administered to patients of any age and for any surgical operation, with the patient remaining ignorant of the physical trauma. However, there are significant dangers of circulatory and respiratory depression, postoperative nausea and vomiting, and changes in thermoregulation.

Regional Anesthesia

Regional anesthesia occurs when an anesthetic substance is given close to a nerve or nerve route at or near the surgical site, thereby preventing the transmission of sensory impulses to central nervous system receptors. The patient undergoing localized anesthesia remains conscious but loses sensation in a specific bodily region. In some cases, loss of reflexes may also occur. A regional anesthetic may be chosen for a variety of surgical procedures and patients, but it is particularly useful for lowering postoperative discomfort, bowel dysfunction, and length of hospital stay in elderly patients.

RThe regional anesthetic can be administered via main nerve blocks or spinal (subdural) blocks, caudal blocks, or epidural blocks.

- Nerve blocks are performed by injecting a local anesthetic around a nerve trunk that supplies the surgical site, such as the jaw, face, or extremities. The onset and duration of the paralysis are determined by the anesthetic agent, its concentration, the volume injected, and the addition of epinephrine, which lengthens the paralysis.
- Local anesthetic injected through a lumbar puncture into the subarachnoid space induces sensory, motor, and autonomic blocking, resulting in spinal anesthesia. This form of anesthetic is utilized for lower abdominal, perineal, and leg surgery. Hypotension, headache, and urinary retention are possible side effects of spinal anesthesia.
- Caudal anesthesia is the injection of local anesthetic into the epidural space through the caudal canal in the sacrum; it may be used for procedures on the lower extremities or perineum.
- Epidural anesthesia is the injection of anesthetic through the intervertebral spaces, typically in the lumbar region (although it may also be used in the thoracic or cervical regions). It is utilized for arm, shoulder, chest, abdomen, pelvis, and leg procedures.

KEYWORD

Epidural block is a numbing medicine given by injection (shot) in a specific place in the back.

Topical and Local Anesthesia

Mucous membranes, open skin, lesions, and burns are treated with topical anesthetic. The most widely utilized agent is a 4% to 10% solution of cocaine, followed by lidocaine and bupivacaine. Anesthetics used topically may be sprayed, distributed, or applied with drug-impregnated gauze or cotton-tipped applicators.

Local anesthesia is the injection of an anesthetic substance, such as lidocaine, bupivacaine, or tetracaine, into a specific body region. The surgeon administers it for modest, brief surgical or diagnostic operations, such as a biopsy. It bathes the tissue surrounding a targeted nerve or infiltrates the tissue beneath the surgical site. Mixing epinephrine with a topical anesthetic helps reduce bleeding by constricting local blood vessels. It also aids in prolonging the duration of analgesia by trapping the anesthetic in the tissue due to the vasoconstriction of the surrounding blood vessels. During general anesthetic operations, local anesthetic may also be given to prolong pain relief after the general anesthetic wears off.

Moderate Sedation/Analgesia

Moderate sedation/analgesia, also known as conscious or procedural sedation, is utilized for minimally invasive and brief procedures. The patient maintains cardiorespiratory function and is able to respond to verbal orders while intravenous delivery of sedatives and analgesics increases the pain threshold, alters the patient's mood, and induces some forgetfulness. The patient retains the capacity to maintain an open airway and is able to respond appropriately. Typically, this type of anesthesia is administered by a perioperative, endoscopy, interventional radiology, or interventional cardiology nurse with specialized training and competency in administering the medications and monitoring the patient's cardiac rate and rhythm, respiratory rate, oxygen saturation, level of consciousness, level of pain, blood pressure, and skin condition.

Informed Consent and Advance Directives

Informed consent is the patient's free agreement to undertake a certain technique or treatment (such as surgery) after receiving the following information, which should be communicated in understandable language (layman's terms) by the physician performing the process or treatment:

- Description of the surgery or treatment, as well as viable alternative treatments
- The underlying pathophysiology and natural history of the condition
- The name and credentials of the person performing the procedure or treatment
- An explanation of the risks involved, including the risk of damage, disfigurement, or death, and the frequency with which they occur
- An explanation that the patient has the right to refuse treatment and that consent can be withdrawn
- Explanation of intended outcome, rehabilitation, and recovery strategy and course

Consent with knowledge protects the patient, practitioner, and healthcare institution. The signed form is both a legal document and an ethical requirement. The individual who will execute the surgery is accountable for obtaining the patient's informed permission. Typically, this is the physician. The nurse may sign as a witness to indicate that the patient signed the permission form voluntarily and with full awareness. The patient has the right to refuse treatment at all times.

If the patient is disoriented, asleep, sedated, mentally incompetent, or a minor, the consent form is invalid (as determined by state laws). In these cases, consent may be given by a parent, spouse, next of kin, or legal guardian. Most states maintain a list of authorized next of kin who are prioritized for signing operating consents. In the event that a question occurs, it is essential to know who is authorized so that the appropriate person may be called. In emergency instances, a physician may get consent through telephone or court order.

TIPS

A do-not-resuscitate order, or DNR order, is a medical order written by a doctor. It instructs health care providers not to do cardiopulmonary resuscitation (CPR) if a patient's breathing stops or if the patient's heart stops beating.

Advance directives, which are also legal documents, allow the patient to establish postoperative healthcare treatment instructions in the event that he or she is unable to communicate these preferences. This permits the patient to share his or her surgical preferences with family members prior to the procedure. Living wills and durable powers of attorney for healthcare are two frequent types of advance directives. The family is aware of the patient's preferences about termination of treatment, resuscitative efforts, and end-of-life decisions in the event that the patient experiences a major, life-threatening complication, such as intraoperative cardiac arrest. Prior to surgery, it is essential to discuss and record the patient's and family's precise preferences, particularly in regards to resuscitation (do-not-resuscitate [DNR]).

Outpatient/Same-day Surgery

As the healthcare system has decreased the length of hospital stays in an effort to cut healthcare expenses, outpatient or same-day (also known as ambulatory) surgical operations have grown more prevalent. These surgical environments can be found in standalone units, hospitals, and doctors' offices. Some standalone surgery centers are specialized in orthopedics or hernia repair, for example. Others conduct a vast array of surgical operations, including major surgical procedures that previously necessitated a three-week hospital stay.

Patients are often admitted to the healthcare facility the morning of surgery. Allowing the patient to spend the night before surgery at home and to recover at home removes a significant amount of the anxiety connected with surgery. Patients who are elderly, chronically ill, or who lack the support networks or finances to offer the necessary postoperative care may require further education and referral to home care agencies.

THE NURSING PROCESS FOR PREOPERATIVE CARE

Patients requiring surgical intervention and nursing care enter the healthcare sector under a range of circumstances, ranging from essentially healthy individuals undergoing planned elective procedures to emergency admissions for treatment of trauma or serious illness (such as a cardiac arrest or stroke). Patients undergoing surgery might be of any age and at any point along the spectrum of health and sickness. It is the role of the nurse to identify factors that influence the risk of a surgical procedure. This includes assessing the physical and emotional needs of the patient and family and developing a care plan based on the correct nursing diagnoses. As the patient advances through the perioperative phase, interventions are aimed to fulfill his or her needs and assist recovery. Some of the desired outcomes that frame the plan of care for the surgical patient, state that the patient will meet the following goals:

- Be free from injury and adverse effects related to positioning, retained foreign objects, or chemical, physical, or electrical hazards
- Be free from infection
- Maintain fluid and electrolyte balance and skin integrity
- Maintain normal body temperature
- Be free from deep vein thrombosis (DVT, formation of a blood clot ["thrombus"] in a deep vein)
- Have their pain managed
- Demonstrate an understanding of the physiologic and psychological responses to the planned surgery
- Participate in a rehabilitation process following surgery

Remember

Perioperative nurses may perform several roles depending on the country they practice in, including circulating, instrument (or scrub) nurse, preoperative (or patient reception) nurse, Post Anaesthetic Care Unit or recovery nurse, registered nurse first assistant (RNFA), and patient educator.

Assessing

The significance of preoperative evaluation cannot be overstated. Preoperative examinations uncover factors that may place the patient at a higher risk for complications during and after surgery.

Assessment of the surgical patient includes:

- Obtaining a health history and performing a physical assessment to establish a baseline database
- Identifying risk factors and allergies that could pose surgical complications
- Identifying medications and treatments the patient is currently receiving
- Determining the teaching and psychosocial needs of the patient and family
- Determining postsurgical support and referral needs for recovery

The assessment is often performed several days before surgery as part of preoperative laboratory screening and teaching; this is referred to as preadmission testing. It could occur in a hospital, surgical clinic, office, or the patient's home.

Patients undergoing outpatient or same-day surgery are required to undergo intensive preoperative tests and education by nurses. Frequently, preoperative education is reinforced with preoperative screening tests, which are normally administered within 30 days of the anticipated surgery. As part of the preoperative evaluation and education for outpatient/same-day surgery, the patient and their family are instructed.

KEYWORD

Psychosocial status refers to the combination of psychological and social factors that influence an individual's overall well-being and functioning. It encompasses aspects of a person's mental, emotional, and social state, including their thoughts, feelings, behaviors, relationships, and social support systems.

Health History

The health history helps the nurse personalize the preoperative assessment by identifying risk factors and strengths in the patient's physical and psychosocial status. Health history information pertinent to the surgical experience includes the patient's developmental level, medical history, medications, previous surgeries, perceptions and knowledge of the upcoming surgery, nutrition, use of alcohol, illicit drugs or nicotine, activities of daily living and occupation, coping patterns, and support and sociocultural needs.

Developmental Considerations

Surgery poses a larger danger to infants and older individuals than to children and young or middle-aged adults. Because of the infant's smaller total blood volume, even a modest loss of blood is cause for concern due to the possibility of dehydration and failure to respond to the surgical need for extra oxygen. In addition, the airway is small, soft, and flexible, and newborns and young children are prone to upper respiratory infections, such as colds, which can lead to airway blockage and hypoxia. This population is susceptible to developing bronchospasm, stridor, and respiratory arrest rapidly. On the day of surgery, if a child exhibits signs of even moderate respiratory illnesses, the procedure will be postponed until the infection has resolved.

Because the infant's shivering reflex has not fully developed, hypothermia and hyperthermia are more likely to occur after surgery. Their decreased glomerular filtration rate and creatinine clearance can impede the metabolism of medicines requiring renal biotransformation. Due to the immaturity of the liver during the first year of life, muscle relaxants and opioids may have extended effects.

KEYWORD

Bronchospasm occurs when the muscles that line the airways of the lungs constrict or tighten, reducing airflow by 15 percent or more.

Aging-related physiological changes enhance the surgical risk for elderly patients. These changes reduce the ability of older individuals to respond to the stress of surgery, modify the effects of preoperative and postoperative drugs and anesthesia, and prolong or alter the wound healing process. With an aging population, monitoring physiologic changes is essential for providing older surgery patients with informed, safe, and holistic nursing care. Chronic illnesses, which are more prevalent in the elderly population, increase surgical risk and may necessitate modifications to standard perioperative treatments. For instance, a patient with congestive failure may be more easily exhausted and, as a result, unable to recover after surgery as quickly.

Medical History

The medical history contains details regarding past and present ailments. Pathologic alterations resulting from past and present diseases increase surgical risk and the chance of postoperative complications. Preoperative examinations and documentation are required to create a database for tailored intraoperative and postoperative assessments and interventions. The following are examples of diseases and associated risks:

- Cardiovascular disorders, including thrombocytopenia, hemophilia, recent myocardial infarction or cardiac surgery, heart failure, and dysrhythmias, increase the risk for bleeding and hypovolemic shock, hypotension, venous stasis, thrombophlebitis, and overhydration with intravenous fluids.

- Respiratory problems such as pneumonia, bronchitis, asthma, emphysema, and chronic obstructive pulmonary disease increase the risk for respiratory depression from anesthesia as well as postoperative pneumonia, atelectasis, and changes in acid–base balance.
- Kidney and liver problems affect the patient's anesthetic response, fluid and electrolyte balance, acid–base balance, drug metabolism and excretion, and wound healing.
- Endocrine illnesses, particularly diabetes, raise the risk of hypoglycemia or acidosis, impede wound healing, and increase the risk of postoperative cardiovascular issues.

KEYWORD

Respiratory depression happens when the lungs fail to exchange carbon dioxide and oxygen efficiently.

Medications

The use of prescribed, over-the-counter, or herbal medications can change the patient's reaction to the stress of surgery and the effects of the anesthetic agent and enhance the associated risk. Some herbal products can promote bleeding, while others may enhance the effects of anesthetics that suppress respiration. Surgical risk is increased by drugs in the following categories:

- Anticoagulants (may precipitate hemorrhage)
- Diuretics (may cause electrolyte imbalances, with resulting respiratory depression from anesthesia)
- Tranquilizers (may increase the hypotensive effect of anesthetic agents)
- Adrenal steroids (abrupt withdrawal may cause cardiovascular collapse in long-term users)
- Antibiotics in the mycin group (when combined with certain muscle relaxants used during surgery, may cause respiratory paralysis)
- Oral antidiabetic medications (such as metformin hydrochloride) may react with radiologic (x-ray) iodinated contrast dyes, and cause acute renal failure

Many medications are discontinued before the surgery, but the nurse should know the purposes and actions of the patient's drugs as well as the physician's orders. Specific medications may be given on the morning of surgery with sips of water (e.g., patients with heart or cardiovascular problems or diabetes mellitus).

Previous Surgery

In order to address the patient's physical and psychological demands during the perioperative phase, it is essential to have information regarding previous surgical procedures. Physical ramifications of prior surgical procedures are crucial to the intraoperative and postoperative stages (e.g., previous heart or lung surgery may necessitate adaptations in anesthesia and in positioning during surgery). Prior complications, such as malignant hyperthermia, latex sensitivity, pneumonia, thrombophlebitis, or surgical site infection, may place the patient at risk during the current procedure, demanding individualized postoperative surveillance.

The patient's prior surgical experiences influence the preoperative treatment strategy, particularly if they were poor. When the interview evokes negative views regarding the surgical experience, pain management, or nurse measures performed to avert complications after previous procedures, the need of training and joint goal setting increases. For children, the admission process, blood testing, injections, the time before and during transit to the operating room, and the recovery period in PACU are the most stressful events preceding surgery.

In addition to past surgical experiences, the patient's views and understanding about the upcoming procedure should be evaluated. When preparing a patient for surgery, organizing patient and family education, and preparing for discharge, it is crucial to address the patient's psychological and familial requirements based on his or her inquiries or statements on the surgery.

KEYWORD

Gastroesophageal reflux disease (GERD) is a condition in which the stomach contents leak backward from the stomach into the esophagus (food pipe).

Nutritional Status

Both malnutrition and obesity increase the chance of surgical complications. Surgical procedures raise the body's nutritional requirements for normal tissue repair and infection resistance. A malnourished patient is more susceptible to fluid and electrolyte imbalance changes, delayed wound healing, and wound infection. Patients who are obese are more susceptible to respiratory, cardiovascular, positional damage, deep vein thrombosis, and gastrointestinal issues. Patients who are overweight may suffer from obstructive sleep apnea, putting them at risk for diminished respiratory function. They may also be suffering from gastroesophageal reflux disease (GERD), which puts them at risk for aspiration of stomach contents. Therefore, postoperative problems such as delayed wound healing, wound infection, and disruption of the wound's integrity are more prevalent in patients with fatty tissue.

Use of Alcohol, Illicit Drugs, or Nicotine

Alcoholic patients require larger dosages of anesthetic agents and postoperative analgesics, which increases the risk for drug-related problems. Patients who utilize illegal drugs are at risk for anesthetic drug interactions. These should be noted in the medical record for safe anesthetic treatment, as they are unique to the illicit drug administered. The use of intravenous drugs may cause veins to become rigid, irritated, and unsuitable for anesthetic drug administration.

Patients who smoke have an increased chance of developing respiratory problems following surgery. All patients retain pulmonary secretions during anesthesia, but smokers, who have higher mucous secretions and less ciliary action in the tracheobronchial tree, have more difficulty clearing the airways after surgery. Moreover, the tracheobronchial mucosa of smokers is persistently irritated, and anesthesia exacerbates this irritation. Hypoxia and postoperative pneumonia are risks for patients who smoke. Smoking hinders the healing of wounds by restricting blood vessels and reducing blood flow to the healing tissues.

KEYWORD

Hypoxia is a state in which oxygen is not available in sufficient amounts at the tissue level to maintain adequate homeostasis; this can result from inadequate oxygen delivery to the tissues either due to low blood supply or low oxygen content in the blood (hypoxemia).

Activities of Daily Living and Occupation

Habits of physical activity, rest, and sleep are essential for reducing postoperative problems and improving recovery. A patient with an established exercise routine has better cardiovascular, pulmonary, metabolic, and musculoskeletal performance, hence decreasing surgical risks. Rest and sleep are necessary for physical and mental adaptation and recuperation following surgical stress. The nurse is able to customize interventions to encourage rest and sleep based on the patient's medical history.

Numerous surgical treatments necessitate a postponement of the patient's return to a career or occupation or may influence the patient's ability to make a living. The nurse is better able to plan appropriate instruction and referrals when she is aware of a patient's typical occupation and worries about returning to work.

Coping Patterns and Support Systems

Assessing the patient's psychological, social, and spiritual components is as crucial as obtaining a physical history and conducting a physical examination. Surgery is a significant source of psychological stress that impacts coping strategies, support networks, and unique human needs. Whether planned or unplanned, significant or tiny, a surgical procedure creates worry and fear. During the health history assessment, the nurse can take signals from the patient's and family's verbal and nonverbal communication to identify anxieties and concerns and design nursing interventions to offer the essential knowledge and emotional support for a successful surgical recovery.

KEYWORD

Postoperative agony refers to severe and distressing pain experienced by individuals after undergoing surgery.

Surgery is an unknown event over which an individual has little control; the resulting anxiety and worry can manifest in a variety of ways, including anger, retreat, indifference, confrontation, and questioning. Patients frequently dread the unknown, suffering or death, and alterations to their physical image and sense of self. Typically, the patient is anxious about the surgery itself, including the anesthetic, the diagnosis, the future, financial and familial responsibilities, pain tolerance, and the possibility of disfigurement or handicap. Fears that the anesthesia will not "put me to sleep," that the patient will die during surgery, or that he or she would be unable to tolerate postoperative agony are common. Surgical procedures frequently result in lasting adjustments to the patient's body structure, function, or appearance, causing patients to dread alterations to their physical attractiveness, social interactions, and sexuality.

The establishment of a trusting nurse–patient connection, which is vital for identifying and resolving fear, requires therapeutic communication skills. Encourage the patient to identify and articulate their anxieties; conversing about fears can typically decrease their intensity. Concurrently, inaccurate knowledge can be discovered and corrected, strengths can be identified, and instruction can be administered. Fear reduction is crucial for preoperative preparation; the addition of mental stress to the physical stress of surgery increases surgical risk. The nursing history should elicit the patient's coping mechanisms for stress reduction.

The support systems identified in the assessment phase of preoperative nursing care might facilitate stress management. Family members or significant others should be included as much as possible in the initial interview and discussions of anxieties and concerns. Encourage family members to offer assistance prior to and following surgical procedures. Encourage parents to accompany their child to the preoperative waiting area and to the recovery area once the youngster is awake, if allowed.

KEYWORD

Surgical interventions are performed by trained surgeons or surgical teams in specialized healthcare settings such as hospitals or surgical centers.

Identifying the patient's spiritual beliefs facilitates the fulfillment of his or her spiritual requirements. Acceptance, participation in prayer or other rituals, and/or referral to a spiritual leader can fulfill these requirements. Faith in a higher being or source of personal strength gives many individuals with support and helps to alleviate their concerns.

Additionally, the necessity for additional support systems might be determined during the initial interview. A patient undergoing a colostomy, heart transplant, or mastectomy, for instance, could benefit from a preoperative visit from a person who has undergone the same procedure and successfully adapted.

Sociocultural Needs

Individual factors, such as family health beliefs and practices, economic concerns, and cultural/ethnic background, influence an individual's views of and reactions to the surgical experience. A patient who requires surgery but was raised in a family that views surgical intervention as the final option for treating sickness may be unwilling to undergo the procedure or may be convinced that he or she will die as a result. This patient's worry may make them more susceptible to surgical danger. Family values and cultural/ethnic identity also have an impact on responses to instruction, physical care, and pain. A male patient raised with the attitude that it is unmanly to admit pain, for instance, may display a stoic acceptance of discomfort and refuse postoperative drugs.

Additionally, cultural and ethnic factors influence the patient's reactions and impressions of the surgical experience. The patient's cultural background may necessitate the individualization of nursing treatments to match their requirements in areas including language, food preferences, family relationships and participation, personal space, and health beliefs and practices. A patient from a culture that views bed rest as the most important therapy for illness or injury, for instance, may find it difficult to accept the need for postoperative exercises and early ambulation.

Physical Assessment

Assessing the patient's current physical condition yields information that can be used to reduce surgical risk and potential postoperative problems.

Various preoperative screening procedures provide objective information regarding normal bodily function. In the event of anomalies, these tests provide information for medical actions to enhance the patient's physical condition and so reduce the chance of surgical problems. The nurse is responsible for ensuring that the patient understands the tests, that adequate specimens are taken, that the results are entered in the patient's record prior to surgery, and that any aberrant findings are reported.

Chest x-rays, electrocardiograms, full blood counts, electrolyte values, and urinalysis are standard preoperative screening procedures. Significant abnormal findings include an elevated white blood cell count (infection), a decreased hematocrit and hemoglobin level (bleeding, anemia), hyperkalemia or hypokalemia (increased risk for cardiac problems), elevated blood urea nitrogen or creatinine levels (possible renal failure), and abnormal urine constituents (indicating infection or fluid imbalances).

Did you get it?

In 1901, Einthoven, working in Leiden, the Netherlands, used the string galvanometer: the first practical ECG.[97] This device was much more sensitive than the capillary electrometer Waller used.

Diagnosing

Nursing diagnoses for patients in the preoperative phase may be outlined for various actual or potential problems for which a patient is at risk. These are produced through the study of subjective and objective data collected from the health history and physical examination, as well as information from other members of the healthcare team and screening tests. Numerous diagnoses represent risk assessment and are established to guide interventions for intraoperative and postoperative patient needs. Nursing care must be consistent and documented throughout the perioperative period. The preoperative nursing diagnosis provides the foundation for consistent, holistic care from admission through recovery.

Outcome Identification and Planning

The length of the preoperative phase affects the preoperative nursing care provided. Patients who reach the hospital through the emergency department and require immediate surgery, as well as those who undergo outpatient/same-day surgery, may not have sufficient time for thorough evaluations and education. In such situations, the nurse must utilize standard preoperative plans and customize them for the specific patient and family. The outcomes for all surgical patients are standardized, but nurse interventions are tailored to meet the priority demands of specific individuals and scenarios.

KEYWORD

Nutritional balance means that you consume just the right amount of calories, macronutrients and micronutrients from your diet.

In the preoperative phase, the nurse, the patient, and the patient's family discuss and agree upon the anticipated outcomes for the entire perioperative period. Specific appropriate outcomes include that the patient: • Is physically and emotionally prepared for surgery; • Demonstrates turning, coughing, and deep-breathing exercises; • Verbally demonstrates an understanding of postoperative pain management; • Maintains adequate fluid intake and nutritional balance to meet needs; and • Maintains adequate fluid intake and nutritional balance to meet needs.

Implementing

The preoperative nursing interventions prepare the patient psychologically and physically for surgery and the postoperative period.

Preparing the Patient Psychologically through Communicating

Surgery is nearly always regarded as a life-threatening emergency and elicits anxiety and panic. By focusing on therapeutic dialogue and patient and family education, nurses can minimize anxiety and facilitate patients' recoveries. Each patient is a unique individual who reacts differently to the surgical procedure. One note of caution: Avoid false reassurance. In an effort to alleviate the patient's concern and fear, the nurse may be inclined to reassure him or her that everything will be alright. Such a response denies the patient's emotional needs, stifles therapeutic communication and erodes trust, and may be false.

Preparing the Patient Psychologically Through Teaching

In the preoperative phase, the nursing role of educating patients about postoperative activities is carried out. Patients and their families must be informed about surgical events and sensations, pain management, and the physical exercises required to reduce the risk of postoperative problems and aid recovery. The teaching–learning process is customized to satisfy both common and unique patient requirements. Timing, the individual patient and his or her support system, the type of surgery, and group versus individual sessions affect the success of preoperative instruction. It has been demonstrated that preoperative education reduces postoperative complications and length of stay, and positively influences recovery. Patients who have received thorough preoperative teaching do better throughout surgery and are better equipped to control their pain and engage in appropriate self-care activities.

KEYWORD

Healthcare team is the group of professionals who contribute to your care and treatment as a patient.

The time of teaching is a crucial factor: Teaching too far in advance of surgery or when the patient is anxious is less effective. In the current healthcare system, patients frequently check into the hospital on the day before surgery, necessitating an adjustment to the instructional schedule. Many institutions provide patient education prior to admission in order to prepare them for surgery. Whether performed before or after admission, a preoperative teaching checklist provides nurses with organized and thorough instruction requirements.

TEACHING ABOUT SURGICAL EVENTS AND SENSATIONS

Patients and their families must know when surgery is scheduled, how long the surgery and post anesthesia care will last, and what will be done before and following surgery (e.g., procedures, medications, equipment). If the operation is elective, a tour of the operating room or a video of the preoperative journey may reduce anxiety and fear of the unknown. For children, a tour or video is extremely beneficial. An explanation of surgical events includes a description of the various healthcare team members, where and when to report for admission, instructions for preoperative fasting and bowel prep, if ordered, instructions for taking special medications, and the necessity of bringing a responsible adult to drive the patient home. If a patient has had anesthesia or sedation, he or she is not permitted to drive or take public transportation alone.

Informing patients of the sensory information they may encounter during the perioperative period is also beneficial. Teaching should include information about dry mouth and drowsiness from preoperative medications, a sore throat from the insertion of an endotracheal tube, a gradual return of feeling and movement after spinal anesthesia, and pain from the surgical incision, even though the sensations vary depending on the type of surgery. Patients should also be informed of the room's temperature, the bed's firmness, the noises and sights of several healthcare professionals wearing surgical masks, and the intense overhead lighting. Assure the patient that he or she is the most important individual in the room and that he or she will receive excellent care and comfort.

Teaching about Pain Management

KEYWORD

Pain management is an aspect of medicine and health care involving relief of pain in various dimensions, from acute and simple to chronic and challenging.

Pain is a typical component of surgical procedures and a key concern for patients and their families. Several professional organizations have established guidelines for the management of acute surgical pain based on scientific evidence. The rules are founded on the following tenets: (1) the patient's perception of pain is the determining factor for pain management; (2) pain must be examined as frequently as every two hours after major surgery; and (3) older patients are at risk for both undertreatment and overtreatment of pain. Continued or unresolved discomfort might lengthen a patient's recovery time and delay discharge. Unrelieved postoperative pain should be regarded as a major surgical complication, not as a common occurrence. The nurse is responsible for assessing, implementing, and evaluating a pain management strategy, as well as training the patient preoperatively on how to effectively communicate and report pain. Preoperatively, children can be introduced to an age-appropriate pain scale.

Inform the patient and family that the physician will order and the nurse will deliver pain meds. The physician may prescribe pain drugs to be administered regularly or as needed. If medication is prescribed on an as-needed basis, there is a time limit between doses (e.g., every 2 or 4 hours). The patient must request medicine and should do so before the onset of severe pain. If the medicine fails to alleviate the patient's discomfort or if it causes undesirable side effects (such as nausea and vomiting), a substitute medication may be prescribed. There is a low risk of addiction to pain medicines used for postoperative pain treatment. Utilizing relaxation techniques (such as deep breathing, music, and guided visualization) augments the effectiveness of pain drugs.

Transcutaneous electrical nerve stimulation (TENS), pressure-controlled pain pumps filled with local anesthetics with soaker drains inside the incision, patient-controlled analgesia (PCA), and patient-controlled epidural anesthesia are alternative methods of pain control that may be used after surgery. Before surgery, the patient should be instructed on how to employ these pain management techniques, and their efficacy should be evaluated following surgery.

Teaching about Physical Activities

The most common causes of postoperative complications are alterations in cardiovascular and respiratory function, including atelectasis, pneumonia, thrombophlebitis, and emboli. Breathing deeply, coughing, incentive spirometry, leg exercises, and turning in bed are physical activities that minimize the risk of these problems. These skills are introduced during the preoperative phase. Before undergoing surgery, the patient should be able to describe the purpose and show the tasks.

Remember

Incisional pain is a unique but common form of acute pain. Because effective postoperative analgesia reduces morbidity following surgery, new treatments continue to be sought.

Deep Breathing

During surgery, the cough reflex is inhibited, mucus collects in the tracheobronchial passages, and the lungs are not adequately ventilated. As a result of the anesthetic, pain medications, and incisional pain, postoperative breathing is frequently less effective. Due to incisional pain, patients with thoracic or upper abdominal incisions are particularly susceptible to shallow respiration. As a result, alveoli do not expand and may collapse, and secretions are retained, hence increasing the risk for atelectasis and lung infection. Deep-breathing exercises hyperventilate the alveoli and prevent them from collapsing, enhance lung expansion and volume, aid in expelling anesthetic gases and mucus, and facilitate tissue oxygenation.

Coughing

Coughing helps clear mucus from the respiratory tract and is typically taught alongside deep breathing. Patients with a higher risk for respiratory problems should cough more frequently. Because coughing is frequently uncomfortable, the patient should be instructed on how to splint the incision (i.e., support the incision with a cushion or folded bath towel) and how to make the most of the time following the administration of pain medication.

Incentive Spirometry

Patients undergoing surgery are frequently prescribed an incentive spirometer, and the correct technique should be rehearsed prior to an operation. This device increases lung volume and alveolar expansion while facilitating venous return. A gauge on the incentive spirometry gadget gives an immediate positive reward for the patient's breathing attempts.

Leg Exercises

During surgery, venous blood return from the legs is slowed, and certain surgical postures, such as elevating the legs in the lithotomy position, further reduce venous return. Thrombophlebitis and emboli are potential consequences of circulatory stasis in the legs. Leg workouts promote venous return through quadriceps and gastrocnemius flexion and contraction. Leg exercises must be tailored to each patient's needs, physical condition, doctor's preference, and agency protocol. Figure 7.2 illustrates how to instruct the patient in leg exercises.

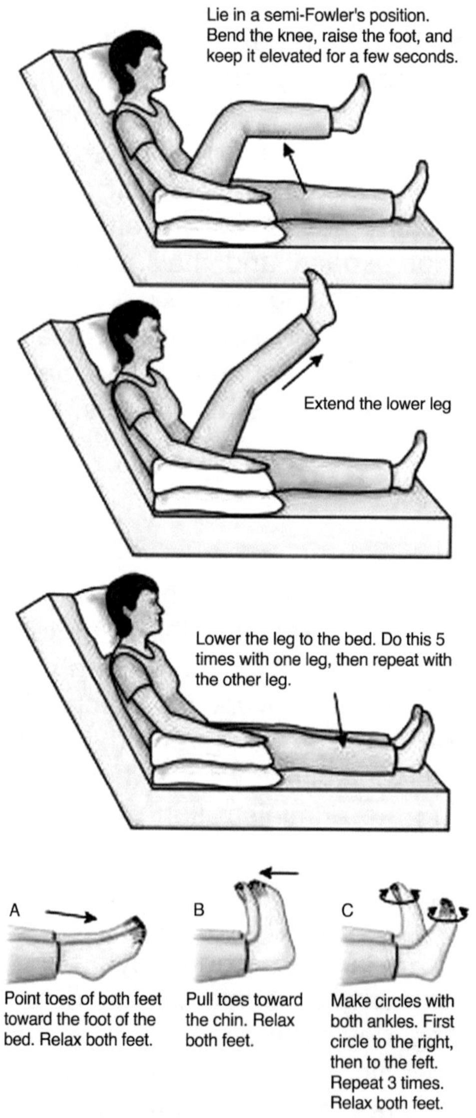

Lie in a semi-Fowler's position. Bend the knee, raise the foot, and keep it elevated for a few seconds.
Extend the lower leg
Lower the leg to the bed. Do this 5 times with one leg, then repeat with the other leg.
A
B
C
Point toes of both feet toward the foot of the bed. Relax both feet.
Pull toes toward the chin. Relax both feet.
Make circles with both ankles. First circle to the right, then to the feft. Repeat 3 times. Relax both feet.

Figure 7.2. Leg exercises to increase venous return.

Turning in Bed

Turning in bed promotes venous return, pulmonary function, and intestinal peristalsis and prevents unrelieved skin pressure, which would occur if the patient remained in a single position. Although turning in bed sounds simple, incisional pain makes it challenging, highlighting the necessity to practice it prior to surgery. To turn in bed, the patient should elevate one knee, hold the side rail on the side toward which he or she is moving, and roll over while pushing with the bent leg and pulling on the side rail. While turning, a little pillow is useful for splinting the wound. When awake, the patient should shift and change positions in bed every two hours.

Remember

The circulating nurse observes for breaches in surgical asepsis and coordinates the needs of the surgical team. The circulating nurse is not scrubbed in the case but rather manages the care and environment during surgery.

Preparing the Patient Physically

Physical preparation for surgery varies according to the patient's physical condition and unique needs, the type of surgery, and the physician's prescriptions. Certain nursing treatments in the areas of cleanliness and skin preparation, elimination, nutrition and fluids, and rest and sleep are recommended for all surgical patients. Additionally, the nurse is responsible for the patient's preparation and safety on the day of operation.

Hygiene and Skin Preparation

The skin is the body's first line of protection against microbes, and surgical incisions present an opportunity for infection. Therefore, the skin is prepped to reduce the risk of postoperative surgical site infection and limit skin contamination.

At the surgical site, an antibacterial soap or solution is used to eliminate microorganisms from the skin. The patient can perform this while bathing or showering. A shower should ideally be taken the night before and/or the morning of surgery. Children and adults can be bathed preoperatively with microfiber towels saturated with chlorhexidine gluconate antimicrobial skin antiseptic, which kills skin germs and leaves an antimicrobial film on the skin to prevent surgical site infections. Additionally, shampooing the hair and cleaning the fingernails lower the amount of organisms on the body.

Before undergoing surgery, it may be required to shave the operative site. However, the necessity for hair removal is contingent on the quantity of hair, the location of the incision, and the type of surgical treatment being performed. This may be performed on the unit or in the operating room just prior to the surgery, typically in the surgical holding area. If hair must be removed, AORN recommends using hair clippers, rather than shaving the area, as was done in the past (see the accompanying box, PICO in Practice: Asking Clinical Questions). Shaving should be performed as soon to the time of operation as possible if the surgeon requires it. In the patient record, the condition of the skin and the method of hair removal and skin preparation must be mentioned.

KEYWORD

Surgical treatment can range from minor procedures performed in outpatient settings to complex surgeries requiring hospitalization and specialized surgical teams.

Elimination

Emptying the bowel of feces prior to surgery is no longer a standard technique, but the nurse must use preoperative assessments to evaluate if an order to promote bowel elimination is necessary. If the patient has not had a bowel movement for several days or has undergone barium diagnostic testing prior to surgery, an enema is used to prevent postoperative constipation.

Whenever a patient is scheduled for surgery of the gastrointestinal tract, a bowel prep and a cleansing enema are typically administered. Peristalsis does not resume until 24 to 48 hours after bowel manipulation; hence, preoperative washing aids in reducing postoperative constipation. Having an empty intestine also prevents contamination of the surgical region.

In order to prevent bladder distention or inadvertent harm, an indwelling urine catheter may be inserted prior to surgery, particularly for patients undergoing pelvic surgery. If there is no indwelling catheter, the patient should void immediately prior to receiving preoperative medications to ensure a bladder that is empty during surgery.

Nutrition and Fluids

To counteract fluid, blood, and electrolyte loss during surgery and to assist in anesthetic administration and tissue regeneration after surgery, patients must be sufficiently nourished and hydrated prior to surgery. Assessments performed before a surgery establish a baseline for physical preparation, including the requirement for extra nourishment, fluids, or electrolytes. A malnourished patient may require parenteral nutrition and intravenous electrolyte supplementation. If the patient's screening tests reveal a hemoglobin level of less than 10 g/dL and a hematocrit of less than 33%, blood or blood component therapy may be administered prior to surgery to maintain volume and improve tissue oxygenation. The American Society of Anesthesiologists (1999) changed the practice standards for preoperative fasting. For many years, maintaining a nothing by mouth (NPO) status for at least eight hours prior to surgery was the standard. The diet depends on the type of surgery and anesthesia that will be administered. Patients are permitted to consume liquids or food up to two hours before surgery, depending on the type of surgery and with physician approval. If clear drinks are permitted, they must be precisely defined for the patient and include water, fruit juices without pulp, fizzy beverages, clear tea, and black coffee. Patients, particularly children, may be less frightened, better hydrated, and have fewer headaches and nausea after surgery if they are permitted to consume certain fluids (including breast milk for newborns) up to 2 to 4 hours before the operation. Patients undergoing a colonoscopy should refrain from eating prepared foods containing the synthetic fat dietary ingredient Olestra, which is used in potato chips. This substance is not usually removed completely from the intestines and causes yellow, sticky plaques to develop on colonoscopes and surgical instruments. It may also cover lesions of mucosal tissue.

KEYWORD

Oxygenation refers to the process of providing oxygen to the body's tissues and cells. It is a vital function necessary for the proper functioning of various organs and systems.

The nurse explains the reason for NPO to the patient and, at the appropriate time, removes all food and fluids from the patient's bedside and places a sign above the patient's bed so that other members of the health care team and visitors are aware of the restriction. The physician should be alerted immediately if the patient consumes food or liquid, as the procedure may be postponed or canceled.

Rest and Sleep

Rest and sleep are essential for lowering stress prior to surgery and promoting healing and recovery following surgery. For hospitalized surgical patients, the nurse can facilitate rest and sleep in the immediate preoperative period by addressing psychological needs, teaching, providing a quiet environment, encouraging relaxation or comfort measures that are personally effective, or administering the prescribed bedtime sedative medication.

Preparing the Patient on the Day of Surgery

Often, a preoperative checklist is used to specify the nurse's duties on the day of surgery; these actions must be done and documented before the patient is transferred to the operating room. Some of these actions have been described previously (e.g., NPO, preoperative teaching, informed consent, skin preparation, screening tests, bladder elimination).

The following drugs may be administered prior to surgery:

- Sedatives, such as diazepam (Valium), midazolam (Versed), or lorazepam (Ativan) to alleviate anxiety and decrease recall of events related to surgery
- Anticholinergics, such as atropine and glycopyrrolate (Robinul), to decrease pulmonary and oral secretions and to prevent laryngospasm
- Narcotic analgesics, such as morphine and meperidine hydrochloride (Demerol), to facilitate patient sedation and relaxation and to decrease the amount of anesthetic agent needed
- Neuroleptanalgesic agents, such as fentanyl citratedroperidol (Innovar), to cause a general state of calmness and sleepiness
- Histamine-2 receptor blockers, such as cimetidine (Tagamet) and ranitidine (Zantac), to decrease gastric acidity and volume

REVIEW QUESTIONS

1. What are the phases of the perioperative period?
2. Explain the surgical procedure classification.
3. Describe the nursing process for preoperative care.
4. Discuss the teaching about pain management.
5. What are the physical activities during surgery?

MULTIPLE CHOICE QUESTIONS

1. The nurse is preparing Mrs. Ogg for surgery for treatment of a ruptured spleen as the result of an automobile crash. The nurse knows that this type of surgery belongs in which of the following categories?

a. Minor, diagnostic
b. Minor, elective
c. Major, emergency
d. Major, palliative

2. A nurse has been asked to witness a patient's signature on an informed consent form for surgery. For which one of these patients would the document be valid?

a. A 92-year-old patient who is severely confused
b. A 45-year-old patient who is oriented and alert
c. A 10-year-old patient who is oriented and alert
d. A 36-year-old patient who has had a narcotic premedication

3. A 72-year-old woman is taking several medications on a regular basis. Which of the following categories of drugs would be most likely to increase her surgical risk?

a. Anticoagulants
b. Antacids
c. Laxatives
d. Sedatives

4. A nurse is caring for an obese patient who has surgery. The nurse monitors this patient for which of the following postoperative complications?

a. Hunger
b. Impaired wound healing
c. Hemorrhage
d. Gas pains

5. A nurse is teaching a man scheduled to have same day surgery. Which teaching method would be most effective in preoperative teaching for ambulatory surgery?

a. Lecture

b. Discussion

c. Audiovisuals

d. Written instructions

Answers to Multiple Choice Questions

1. (c) 2. (b) 3. (a) 4.(b) 5. (d)

REFERENCES

1. Algren, C. L., &Arnow, D. (2007). Pediatric variations of nursing interventions. In M. J. Hockenberry& D. Wilson (Eds.), Wong's nursing care of infants and children, (8th ed.) (pp. 1083–1139). St. Louis: Saunders Elsevier.
2. American Society of Anesthesiologists, Inc. (1999). Practice guidelines for preoperative fasting and the use of pharmacologic agents to reduce the risk of pulmonary aspiration: Application to healthy patients undergoing elective procedures. Anesthesiology, 90, 896–905.
3. American Society of PeriAnesthesia Nurses (ASPAN). (2008). Standards of perianesthesia nursing practice. Thorofare, NJ: American Society of PeriAnesthesia Nurses.
4. Association of periOperative Registered Nurses (AORN). (2006a). Perioperative patient focused model. Standards, recommended practices, and guidelines. Denver: AORN, Inc.
5. Association of periOperative Registered Nurses (AORN). (2006b). AORN's age-specific competency series. Denver: AORN, Inc.
6. Association of periOperative Registered Nurses (AORN). (2006c). Perioperative patient focused model. In Standards, recommended practices, and guidelines. Denver, CO: Author.
7. Association of periOperative Registered Nurses (AORN). (2008a). Perioperative standards and recommended practices. Denver: AORN, Inc.
8. Association of periOperative Registered Nurses (AORN). (2008b). AORN guidance statement: Postoperative patient care in the ambulatory surgery setting. In Perioperative standards and recommended practices (pp. 219–226). Denver: AORN, Inc.
9. Association of periOperative Registered Nurses (AORN). (2008c). Recommended practices for managing the patient receiving moderate sedation/analgesia. In

Perioperative standards and recommended practices (pp. 461–472). Denver: AORN, Inc.

10. Association of periOperative Registered Nurses (AORN). (2008d). Perioperative patient outcomes. In Perioperative Standards and recommended practices (pp. 37–46). Denver: AORN, Inc.
11. Barash, P. G., Cullen, B. F., &Stoelting, R. K. (2006). Clinical anesthesia (5th ed.). Philadelphia: Lippincott Williams & Wilkins.
12. Cantrel, S. W., Ward, K. S., & Van Wicklen, S. A. (2007). Translating research on venous thromboembolism into practice. AORN Journal, 86(4), 590–602.
13. Clancy, C. M. (2008). The importance of simulation: Preventing hand-off mistakes. AORN Journal, 88(4), 625–627.
14. Crenshaw, J., & Winslow, E. (2002). Preoperative fasting: Old habits die hard. American Journal of Nursing, 102(5), 36–45.
15. DeFazio-Quinn, D. M. (2009). Perianesthesia nursing as a specialty. In C. B. Drain & J. Odon-Forren (Eds.), Perianesthesia nursing: A critical care approach (5th ed.) (pp. 11–31). St. Louis: Saunders Elsevier.
16. DiPaola, C. A. (2008). Preventing deep vein thrombosis: A perioperative nursing imperative. AORN Journal, 88(2), 283–285.
17. Edmiston, C. E., Krepel, C. J., Seabrook, C. R., Lewis, B., Brown, K., & Towne, J. (2008). Preoperative shower revisited: Can high topical antiseptic levels be achieved on the skin surface before surgical admission? Journal of the American College of Surgery, 207(2), 233–239.
18. Hodgson, B. B., &Kizior, R. J. (2007). Saunders nursing drug handbook. St. Louis: Saunders Elsevier.
19. Jacob, E. (2007). Pain assessment and management in children. In Hockenberry, M.J, & Wilson, D. Wong's nursing care of infants and children (8th ed.) (pp. 205–642). St. Louis: Saunders Elsevier.
20. Joint Commission. (2010). National patient safety goals. Available at http://www.jointcommission.org.
21. Nilsson, U. (2008). The anxiety- and pain-reducing effects of music interventions: A systematic review. AORN Journal, 87(4), 780–807.
22. Odom-Forren, J. (2007). Accurate patient handoffs: Imperative for patient safety. Journal of Perianesthesia Nursing, 22(4), 233–234.
23. Patel, N., Bagen, B., Vadera, S., Gil Maltenfort, M., Deutsch, H., Vaccaro, A. A., et al. (2007). Obesity and spine surgery: Relation to perioperative complications. Journal of Neurosurgery and Spine 6(4), 291–297.
24. Pop, R. S., Manworren, R., Guzzetta, C., Hynan, L. (2007). Perianesthesia nurses' pain management after tonsillectomy and adenoidectomy: Pediatric patient outcomes. Journal of Perianesthesia Nursing, 22(2), 91–101.

25. Rothrock, J. (2007). Alexander's care of the patient in surgery (13th ed.). St. Louis: Mosby Elsevier.
26. Susleck, D., Willocks, A., Secrest, J., Norwood, B. K., Holweger, J., Davis, M., et al. (2007). The perianesthesia experience from the patient's perspective. Journal of Perianesthesia Nursing, 22(1), 10–20.

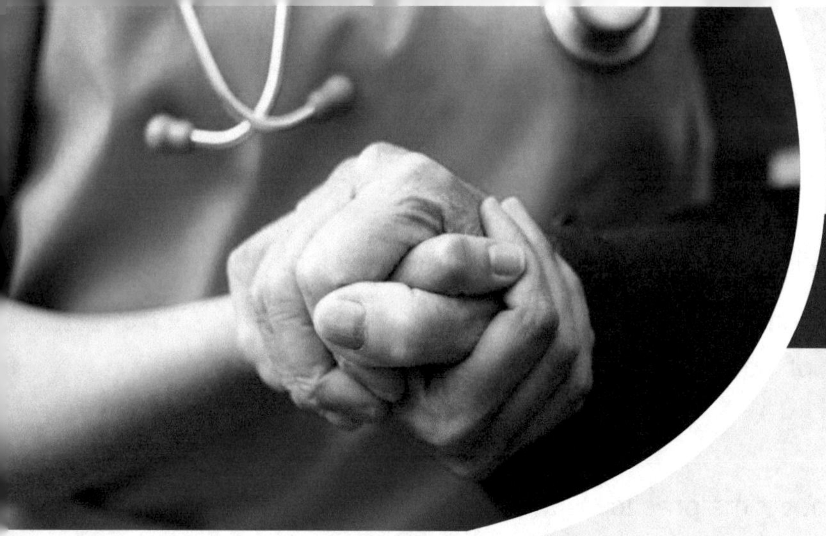

CHAPTER 8

LEGAL AND ETHICAL ASPECTS OF NURSING

"When you're a nurse, you know that every day you will touch a life or a life will touch yours."

—Unknown

INTRODUCTION

Patients are the core of professional and ethical nursing practice. Utilizing and practicing the professional nursing values in the clinical setting might help cause professional, ethical, and legal challenges for nurses. In certain situations, practicing within an ethical context can be difficult. Nurses must make ethical decisions that may present ethical challenges. In planning and delivering safe, high-quality care, nurses make ethical decisions on behalf of the patient. One of the primary tasks of nurses is advocacy. The ethical decision-making of nurses can potentially result in ethical difficulties and legal proceedings. To handle ethical challenges and problems, problem-solving strategies must be employed. In addition, nurses must be familiar with the code of ethics, ethical principles, legal requirements, and regulations that regulate nursing care.

Learning Objectives

After completing the chapter, you will be able to accomplish the following:

- Legal aspects of nursing practice
- Understanding the concept of ethics
- Legal concepts in nursing
- ICN code of ethics
- Measures to prevent the above malpractice situations

Key-Terms

- Nursing regulation
- Legal principles
- Criminal law
- Civil law
- Vicarious liability
- Deontology
- Teleology
- Intuitionism
- Autonomy
- Confidentiality

LEGAL ASPECTS OF THE NURSING PRACTICE

In a democratic society, the legal system provides the foundation for interaction between all segments of the community. It establishes the individual's rights and privileges and provides for the enforcement of rights and reparation of wrongs. All citizens should grasp the laws that regulate their personal and professional life, as well as their legally recognized rights and obligations. It is not acceptable to use ignorance as an excuse for breaking a law. Nurses have legal responsibilities common to all members of the community, and also the responsibilities imposed by the nature of their work, which may be defined as responsibilities in respect of:

- The provision of safe effective nursing care
- The health of the community
- The employing authority
- The nursing profession

KEYWORD

Legislation is the process or result of enrolling, enacting, or promulgating laws by a legislature, parliament, or analogous governing body.

Acts of Parliament

There are, in each state and territory, various Acts, which are laws created by a Parliament. Acts of Parliament are generally referred to as legislation, and they are frequently supplemented by Regulations that provide compliance instructions. As the Acts differ from state to state and territory to territory, nurses are encouraged to familiarize themselves with the Acts applicable to their place of nursing practice.

Common Law

The common law is the body of law created by judges as a result of their judgments in court cases. These precedents (legal principles) can then be applied to similar situations. This body of law is frequently referred to as judge-made law and is just as significant as legislation passed by Parliament. The law of consent and the law of assault and violence are examples.

Types of law

It is essential to understand the differences between criminal and civil law. The scope of criminal law includes offenses against persons and property. The government has the authority to establish minimum standards of acceptable behavior and then strives to control behavior through the police force by enforcing compliance with these norms. A violation of a criminal law is referred to as a crime, and it is punishable by a fine or imprisonment. As offenses against society as a whole, homicide, robbery, rape, and kidnapping are examples of crimes that are viewed as heinous.

KEYWORD

Civil law describe the law that pertains to persons, things, and relationships that develop among them, excluding not only criminal law but also commercial law, labor law, etc.

Civil laws govern the relationships between individuals. Such laws give the instruments for the enforcement of rights and the redress of wrongs. For instance, a person found to have violated civil law is typically forced to pay a sum of money to the individual asserting loss or harm to their person or property. Areas of civil law include trespass, contracts and negligence.

The Employer

An employer, such as a hospital's board of directors, is legally accountable for any acts performed by workers in the course of their employment. This principle of vicarious liability applies to all nurses since it holds an employer liable for the activities of an employee committed in the course of work. While the employer is held liable, they have the right to demand a full financial indemnity from the guilty employee, such as in cases of negligence. An employer must ensure that:

- Employees possess the required qualifications, registration and level of competence
- All legal requirements are met, including valid contracts of employment
- Safety standards are observed in relation to standards of patient care, buildings and equipment

The legal liability of the employer does not absolve a nurse from individual responsibility, and legal action can be taken against a hospital and a nurse or against a nurse as an individual.

Nursing Regulation

Each state and territory in Australia has its own Nurses Act or Health Professions Registration Act and Regulations since the control and regulation of the nursing profession is determined at the state and territory level. Each state and territory has a Nurses Board or Nurses Council constituted of individuals with the authority to register and deregister nurses. Each state or territory Act is broken into sections, with each section addressing a distinct aspect of registration. Due to the fact that each state and territory has its own Act, it is imperative that nurses read the pertinent laws so that they are aware of state and/or territory-specific requirements.

Some states and territories now have a separate registration for midwives, as new education programs make it possible to become a midwife in some jurisdictions by direct entry with a bachelor's degree in midwifery. Additionally, all states and territories have established legislation to safeguard the term "nurse practitioner."

By specifying the conditions under which a nurse may practice in each category of registration, the law safeguards the community by declaring a qualified nurse to be safe and qualified to practice nursing. Nurses who do not meet the requirements of the applicable Nurses or Health Professions Registration Act are not permitted to practice nursing. Currently, a practicing certificate or renewal of registration must be obtained annually from the Nurses Board in each state or territory in order to practice any branch of nursing. The individual nurse is responsible for ensuring that registration or enrollment costs are paid annually.

KEYWORD

Moral reasoning is the study of how people think about right and wrong and how they acquire and apply moral rules.

UNDERSTANDING THE CONCEPT OF ETHICS

Ethics versus Morality

Ethics derives from the Greek term ethos, which means custom or character. Ethics is the branch of philosophy concerned with norms of behavior and moral judgment. It is a method of research that helps individuals comprehend the morality of human behavior. (In other words, it is the study of morals) Ethics, when used in this context, is an activity; it is a method of examining or researching particular concerns concerning human behavior. Ethics refers to the activities or beliefs of a certain group (e.g., the ethics of nurses and physicians). It also refers to the expectations outlined in the organization's code of professional conduct. Ethics concerns what should be, what is right or wrong, and what is good or evil. It is the foundation of moral reasoning and a reflection of a set of ideals. It is a formal process of reasoning used to establish correct behavior. It is stated professionally and openly. An investigation or study of principles and ideals. It is the process of examining and maybe altering one's morals.

Moral: is inclusive of principles and rules of right conduct. It is private or personal. Commitment to principles and values is usually defended in daily life.

Types of Ethics

Did you Know?

In 1847, the American Medical Association adopted its first code of ethics, with this being based in large part upon Percival's work.

- ***Descriptive***: It is the description of the values and beliefs of various cultural, religious or social groups about health and illness.
- ***Normative***: a study of human activities in a broad sense in an attempt to identify human actions that are right or wrong and good and bad qualities. In nursing normative ethics addresses: scope of practice of different categories of nurses and, the level of competence expected.
- ***Analytical***: analyzes the meaning of moral terms. It seeks the reasons why these actions or attitudes are either wrong or right.

Common Ethical Theories

Ethical theories may be compared to lenses that help us to view an ethical problem. Different theories can be useful because they allow us to bring different perspectives into our ethical discussions or deliberations. There are four ethical theories:

- Deontology
- Teleology
- Intuitionism
- The ethics of caring

Deontology (Duty or rule-Based theory)

This theory posits that the rightness or wrongness of an action is determined by the character of the action, rather than by its results. According to this theory, you are acting morally when you adhere to your duties and rights. These moral aspects of existence necessitate accountability. The theory suggests that duties and rights are the proper yardsticks for evaluating behavior. Codes of professional ethics are one location where such factors are given. Such as informed consent and patient respect.

Teleology (utilitarian or end-based theory)

This theory evaluates whether an activity is right or wrong based on its results. According to the utilitarian school of thought, the correct action is the one that has the highest utility or usefulness.

Utilitarians believe that activities are neither good nor terrible in and of themselves; the only variables that make actions good or bad are their outcomes or final results.

Types of Utilitarian Theories

Act utilitarianism: proposes that individuals adopt activities that will, in all circumstances, improve the greater good.

Rule utilitarianism: proposes that individuals select rules that, when consistently followed, increase the overall good.

Intuitions: The belief that humans instinctively know what is right and wrong; that identifying what is right or wrong does not require rational thought or education. For instance, nurses intuitively understand that hitting a client is unethical; this does not require instruction or explanation.

KEYWORD

Accountability is equated with answerability, blameworthiness, liability, and the expectation of account-giving.

The ethic of caring (case based theory)

In contrast to the preceding theories, which are centered on the notion of fairness (justice), ethical caring is founded on relationships. It emphasizes bravery, kindness, dedication, and accountability. Caring is a power that protects and enhances the dignity of the client.

Ethical Principles

Principles are basic ideas that are starting points for understanding and working through a problem. Ethical principles presuppose that nurses should respect the value and uniqueness of persons and consider others to be worthy of high regard. These principles are tents that are important to uphold in all situations. The major principles of nursing ethics are:

- Autonomy
- Beneficence
- Nonmaleficence
- Justice

1. Autonomy

Autonomy is the promotion of independent choice, self-determination and freedom of action. Autonomy means independence and the ability to be self-directed in healthcare. Autonomy is the basis for the client's right to self-determination. It means clients are entitled to make a decision about what will happen to their bodies.

The term autonomy implies for basic elements:

KEYWORD

Autonomy is the ability to make your own decisions about what to do rather than being influenced by someone else or told what to do.

- The autonomous person is respected.
- The autonomous person must be able to determine personal goals. The goals may be explicit or may be less well defined.
- The autonomous person has the capacity to decide on a plan of action. The person must be able to understand the meaning of the choice to be made and deliberate on the various options, while understanding the implications of possible outcomes.
- The autonomous person has the freedom to act upon the choices.

Competent adult clients have the right to consent or refuse treatment even if health care providers do not agree with clients' decisions; their wishes must be respected. However, in most instances, patients are expected to be dependent upon the health care provider. Often times health care professionals are insensitive to ways by which they dehumanize and erode the autonomy of consumers. For example:

- Right after admission patients are asked about personal and private matters.
- Workers who are new to patients may freely enter and leave the patients' room making privacy impossible.

Four factors for violations of patient autonomy:

- Nurses may assume that patients have the same values and goals as themselves.
- Failure to recognize that individuals' thought processes are different.
- Assumptions about patients' knowledge base.
- Focus on work rather than caring.

Infants, young children, people with mental disabilities or incompetence, and comatose patients lack the capacity to participate in health care decision-making. This "surrogate decision maker" would operate on behalf of the client if he or she became unable to make decisions for him or herself.

The autonomy of clients is considered more in the context of broader themes, such as informed consent, paternalism, compliance, and self-determination.

Informed consent: is a process by which patients are informed of the possible outcomes, alternatives and risks of treatments and are required to give their consent freely. It protects the patient's right to autonomy regarding certain treatments and procedures. In particular legal aspects of nursing practice, informed consent will be elaborated upon.

Paternalism is limiting the autonomy of others in order to protect them from seen or predicted harm. The purposeful restriction of another's autonomy that is justified by their needs. Thus, the prevention of any evil or injury is greater than any prospective ills resulting from the interference with an individual's autonomy or freedom. When a patient is deemed incompetent or has limited decision-making capacity, paternalism is appropriate.

Noncompliance: The patient's unwillingness to engage in health care activities. The client's failure to comply with a treatment plan devised by medical professionals. Noncompliance may result from two factors:

- When plans seem unreasonable to the patient
- Patients may be unable to comply with plans for a variety of reasons including resources, lack of knowledge, psychological and cultural factors that are not consistent with the proposed plan of care

2. Beneficence

Benevolence is the act or promotion of good. This is the foundation for all health care practitioners. When nurses deliver pain medicine, conduct a dressing to encourage wound healing, or provide emotional support to a client who is anxious or depressed, they are performing beneficent acts. This principle gives the context and justification for nursing. It creates the foundation for the trust society places in the nursing profession, as well as the trust people place in particular nurses or health care agencies. The principle of beneficence has three components:

- Promote good
- Prevent harm
- Remove evil or harm

KEYWORD

Self-determination is a core principle of international law, arising from customary international law, but also recognized as a general principle of law, and enshrined in a number of international treaties.

3. Nonmaleficence

Nonmaleficence is antithetical to beneficence. It means to refrain from inflicting harm. When working with patients, health care professionals must not inflict harm or suffering. It is to avoid creating intentional harm, the possibility of harm, and harm that arises when performing helpful activities. Example: experimental research with unfavorable effects on the client.

Nonmaleficence also means avoiding harm as a consequence of good. In such cases, the harm must be weighed against the expected benefit.

Remember

Nonmaleficence is the obligation of a physician not to harm the patient. This simply stated principle supports several moral rules – do not kill, do not cause pain or suffering, do not incapacitate, do not cause offense, and do not deprive others of the goods of life.

4. Justice

Justice is fair, equitable and appropriate treatment. It is the foundation of the obligation to serve all clients equally and fairly. A just decision is based on client needs and equitable resource distribution. It would be unreasonable to base such a decision on how much he or she likes each individual client.

5. Veracity

Veracity means telling the truth, which is essential to the integrity of the client-provider relationship

- Health care providers are obliged to be honest with clients.
- The right to self-determination becomes meaningless if the client does not receive accurate, unbiased, and understandable information.

6. Fidelity

Fidelity means being faithful to one's commitments and promises.

- Nurses' commitments to clients include providing safe care and maintaining competence in nursing practice.
- In some instances, a promise is made to a client in an over way.
- Nurse must use good judgment when making promises to client. Fidelity means not only keeping commitment but also keeping or maintaining our obligation.

7. Confidentiality

Confidentiality comes from Latin fide: trust.

- confide as to "show trust by imparting secrets"; "tell in assurance of secrecy"; "entrust; commit to the charge, knowledge or good faith of another"; while
- confidential or in confidence is "a secret or private matter not to be divulged to others"

In the context of health care, confidentiality is the obligation of health professionals (HPs) to maintain the privacy of information received in the course of their work.

Professional standards of ethics (and conduct) frequently include comments regarding maintaining secrecy, however, these declarations are frequently qualified. Confidentiality is the non-disclosure of entrusted private or confidential information. Legally, this responsibility applies to HPs and others, who have access to information about patients, and continues after the patient's death.

Nurses maintain the confidentiality of any information collected in their professional capacity and exercise discretion when disclosing such information. Each nurse will maintain the confidentiality of personal information received in the course of professional duties. The nurse utilizes professional judgment regarding the necessity of disclosing specific details, taking into account the patient's interests, well-being, and safety as well as the legal requirement to reveal some information.

KEYWORD

Professional Standards have been developed with sector professionals and experts to support and inspire your professional learning and career development.

Ethical Arguments for Maintaining Patient Confidentiality

(i) Utilitarian argument

Patients' assurance of privacy increases the likelihood that they will seek therapy (e.g., for complaints that may be personally embarrassing, or related to socially denigrated, or illegal activities, etc.). This ensures that patients are correctly diagnosed and treated. This ultimately contributes to minimizing harm and maximizing good.

(ii) Respect for autonomy (may be a deontological or utilitarian basis) (may be a deontological or utilitarian justification)

Respect for autonomy necessitates allowing individuals to manage the dissemination of their personal information. Such control is necessary for personal liberty (e.g., freedom from compulsion or the ability to pursue one's goals/values).

KEYWORD

Decisional privacy protects the individual from government interference with personal and family decisions."

(iii) Promise keeping

There is an implicit agreement between HPs and patients regarding the confidentiality of patient information. Therefore, a breach of secrecy violates a commitment.

The concept of confidentiality relies on the principle of privacy, which may come from or be conceptually distinct from the concept of autonomy.

Privacy

(1) Bodily privacy

An ethical concept of bodily privacy can be derived from respect for autonomy, where autonomy includes the freedom to decide what happens to one's body.

Bodily privacy is recognized in law: actions in assault, battery and false imprisonment may be available to the person who does not consent to health care.

(2) Decisional privacy

Decisional privacy is distinguished as control over the intimate decisions one makes (e.g., about contraception, abortion, and perhaps health care at the end of one's life).

(3) Informational privacy

This type of privacy underlies the notion of confidentiality.

Arguments for Respecting Privacy

(i) Privacy and property

Personal information is regarded as a kind of property, something one owns.

(ii) Privacy and social relationships

Privacy is a necessary condition for the development and maintenance of relationships, including those between HPs and patients.

(iii) Privacy and the sense of self

The notion that one is a separate self includes the concept of one's body and experiences as one's own. Privacy is to be valued for its role in developing and maintaining our sense of individuation.

KEYWORD

Vulnerability is a weakness that can be exploited by cybercriminals to gain unauthorized access to a computer system.

Limits of Confidentiality

Should the standards of confidentiality always be respected? In certain cases, there are grounds in support of calling into question the absolute necessity of confidentiality. These arguments contain notions associated with the concepts of harm and vulnerability. The harm principle is applicable when a nurse or other expert understands that maintaining confidentiality may result in preventable harm to innocent third parties.

When confidentiality clashes with the duty to warn, the ability to anticipate is a crucial factor to consider. In order to break the concept of confidentiality in favor of a duty to warn, the nurse or other health care provider must be able to rationally foresee danger or injury to an innocent third party.

The harm principle is increased when the vulnerability of the innocent is considered. The obligation to protect others from harm is heightened when the third party is dependent on others or particularly vulnerable. This obligation is known as the vulnerability principle. Vulnerability denotes risk or susceptibility to damage when humans are relatively incapable of defending themselves.

Actions that are deemed ethical are not always deemed lawful. Even while there is an ethical basis for subordinating the principle of secrecy in exceptional circumstances and a legal precedent for doing so, there is a legal risk associated with releasing sensitive information. There is a dynamic tension between the patient's right to privacy and the obligation to warn others. The nurses must know that legal regimes do not always enable careful examination of the ethical consequences of acts.

Disclosure of Information

KEYWORD

Confidentiality involves a set of rules or a promise usually executed through confidentiality agreements that limits the access or places restrictions on certain types of information.

- Disclosure of information is not necessarily an actionable breach of confidence. Disclosure may be allowed, under certain circumstances, when it is requested by: the patient, and where it applies, freedom of information can be used by patients to obtain health care information;
- Other health practitioners (with the patient's consent, and where the information is relevant to the patient's care);
- Relatives in limited circumstances (e.g., parents when it is in the interests of the child);
- Researchers with ethics committee approval (and where the approved process is followed);
- The court;
- The media, if the patient has consented; and
- The police, when the HP has a duty to provide the information.

Unless there is a warrant or a severe crime has been committed, the police are often only given the patient's name, general condition, and injuries. Refer the matter to management and/or seek legal counsel if uncertain. When a patient consents to the release of material to the media, management approval is typically necessary.

Confidentiality is the ethical principle requiring the non-disclosure of private or secret information in which an individual has an interest.

In all circumstances, the standards of health care ethics must be adhered to. The connection between clients and health care providers is governed by rules. The cornerstones of ethical norms are honesty, loyalty, and confidentiality.

Ethical Dilemmas & Ethical Decision Making in Nursing

A dilemma is a scenario in which there are two or more options; it is difficult to establish which option is the best, and the requirements of all those concerned cannot be met by the alternatives. The choices in a dilemma may have both positive and negative characteristics. Ethical challenges in health care encompass questions concerning professional acts and decisions regarding client care. They may cause pain and disagreement among members of the health care team or between doctors and the patient's family.

Models for Ethical Decision-Making

Ethical issues are relevant to everyday living. There is no single solution to such situations. Depending on the persons involved and the event, each circumstance will be unique. However, ethical decision-making models give structures or methods that facilitate reflection on or clarification of an ethical issue. There are numerous models from which to pick, but there is no single optimal technique for making ethical decisions. Models of ethical decision-making are not formulas and do not guarantee that the option you make will be the correct one.

KEYWORD

Personal autonomy is the capacity to decide for oneself and pursue a course of action in one's life, often regardless of any particular moral content.

Model I: A guide to Moral Decision-Making

It outlines a step-by-step process that considers the many aspects of ethical decision-making:

1. Recognizing the moral dimension
   - Is recognizing the decision as one that has moral importance
   - Important clues include conflicts between two or more values or ideals
   - Consider here the levels of ethical guidance in the code of Ethics for registered nurses.
2. Who are the interested parties? What are their relationships?
   - Carefully Identify who has a stake in the decision in this regard, be imaginative and sympathetic.
   - Often there are more parties whose interests should be taken into consideration than is immediately obvious.
   - Look at the relationships between the parties look at their relationship with yourself and with each other, and with relevant institutions.
3. What values are involved?
   - Think through the shared values that are at stake in making this decision.
   - Is there a question of trust? Is personal autonomy a consideration? Is there a question of fairness? Is anyone harmed or helped?
   - Consider your own and others' personal values & ethical principles.

4. Weight the benefits and burdens
   - Benefits might include such things as the production of goods (physical, emotional, financial, and social, etc) for various parties, the satisfaction of preferences and acting in accordance with various relevant valves (such as fairness).
   - Burdens might include causing physical or emotional pain to various parties imposing financial costs and ignoring relevant values.

KEYWORD

Decision making is the process of making choices by identifying a decision, gathering information, and assessing alternative resolutions.

5. Look for analogous cases
   - Can you think of similar decisions? What course of action was taken? Was it a good one? How is the present case like that one? How is it different?
6. Discuss with relevant other
   - The merit of discussion should not be underestimated. Time permitting discuss your decision with as many people as have a take in it.
   - Gather opinions and ask for the reasons behind those opinions.
7. Does this decision according with legal and organizational rules?
   - Some decisions are appropriately based on legal considerations. If an option is illegal, one should think very carefully before thanking that option
   - Discussion may also be affected by organizations of which we are members. For example, the nursing profession has a code of ethics and professional standards that are intended to guide individual decision-making. Institutions may also have policies that limit the options available.

8. *Am I comfortable with this decision? Questions to reflect upon include:*

   - If I carry out this decision, would I be comfortable telling my family about it? My clergy? My mentors?
   - Would I want my children to take my behavior as an example?
   - Is this decision one that a wise, informed, virtuous person would make?
   - Can I live with this decision?

Model 2: Clinical Ethics grid system

This grid system helps construct a summary of the facts that must be considered along with ethical principles to guide ethical decisions in a clinical setting outlined as follows.

1. Medical indications:
    - What is the patient medical problem? History? Diagnosis?
    - Is the problem acute? Chronic? Critical? Emergent? Reversible?
    - What are the goals of treatment etc?
2. Patient preference:
    - What has the patient experienced about preferences for treatment?
    - Has the patient been informed of benefits and risk, understood, and given consent? etc.
3. Quality of life:
    - What are the prospects with or without treatment, for a return to the patient's normal life?
    - Are there biases that might prejudice the provider's evaluation of a patient's quality of life etc?
4. Contextual factors:
    - Are there family issues that might influence treatment decisions?

KEYWORD

Grid systems are aids designers use to build designs, arrange information and make consistent user experiences.

LEGAL CONCEPTS IN NURSING

General Legal Concepts

Law can be defined as those rules made by humans who regulated social conduct in a formally prescribed and legally binding manner. Laws are based upon concerns for fairness and justice.

Functions of Law in Nursing

The law serves a number of functions in nursing:

- It provides a framework for establishing which nursing actions in the care of clients are legal.

- It differentiates the nurse's responsibilities from those of other health professionals.
- It helps establish the boundaries of independent nursing action.
- It assists in maintaining a standard of nursing practice by making nurses accountable under the law.

KEYWORD

Criminal law prescribes conduct perceived as threatening, harmful, or otherwise endangering to the property, health, safety, and welfare of people inclusive of one's self.

Types of Law

Law governs the relationship of private individuals with the government and with each other.

- ***Public Law***: refers to the body of law that deals with relationships between individuals and governmental agencies. An important segment of public law is criminal law which deals with actions against the safety and welfare of public. Examples, theft, homicide, etc.
- ***Private Law or Criminal***: is the body of law that deals with relationships, between individuals. It is categorized as contract law and tort law.
- ***Contract Law***: involves the enforcement of agreements among private individuals or the payment of compensation for failure to fulfill the agreements.
- ***Tort Law***: the word tort means 'wrong " or "bad" in Latin. It defines and enforces duties and rights among private individuals that are not based on contractual agreements. Example of Tort law applicable to nursing
  - Negligence and malpractice
  - Invasion of privacy and assault.

Kinds of Legal Actions

There are two kinds of legal actions:

- Civil or private action.
- Criminal action
- ***Civil actions***: Deals with the relationships between individuals in a society. Example, a man may file a suit against a person who he believes cheated him.
- ***Criminal actions***: Deals with disputes between an individual and the society as a whole. Example if a man shoots a person, society brings him to trial.

Legal Issues in Nursing

Nursing Practice Act: Nursing practice regulations govern nursing practice. Legally define and describe the scope of nursing practice, which the law seeks to regulate, thereby protecting the public as well. It safeguards the user's professional standing. Each nation may have unique laws, but they all have the same purpose: to safeguard the people. It provides the public with a method for ensuring basic criteria for admittance into the profession and identifying unqualified individuals.

KEYWORD

Safeguard is a law, rule, or measure intended to prevent someone or something from being harmed.

Standard of Practice: Through the formation of standard practice, a standard of practice aims to ensure that its practitioners are qualified and safe to practice. An important duty of a professional organization is to establish and implement practice standards. Among the obligations of the profession inherent in creating and implementing standards of practice are the following:

- To establish, maintain, and improve standards
- To hold members accountable for using standards.
- To educate the public to appreciate the standard
- To protect the public from individuals who have not attended the standards or willfully do not follow them and
- To safeguard individual members of the profession.

Standard of nursing practice requires:

- The helping relationship be the nature of client-nurse interaction
- Nurse to fulfill professional responsibilities
- Effective use of the nursing process

Standards of nursing practice are to describe the responsibilities for which nurses are accountable. The standards:

- Reflect the values and practices of the nursing profession
- Provide direction for professional nursing practice.
- Provide a framework for the evaluation of nursing practice
- Defines the profession's accountability to the public and the client outcomes for which nurses are responsible.

In contrast to the functions of other health workers, nursing standards accurately reflect the unique functions and activities performed by nurses.

When professional practice standards are applied, they serve as measuring sticks for licensing, certification, accreditations, quality assurance, peer review, and public policy.

The profession maintains practice standards in part by requiring acceptable entry.

KEYWORD

Mental health encompasses emotional, psychological, and social well-being, influencing cognition, perception, and behavior.

Credentialing

Credentialing is the process of determining and maintaining competence-nursing practice. Credentials include:

- Licensure
- Registration
- Certification
- Accreditation

Licensure: It is a legal permit a government agency grants to individuals to engage in the practice of a profession and to use a particular title. It generally meets three criteria:

- There is a need to protect the public's safety or welfare.
- The occupation is clearly delineated with a separate, distinct area of work
- There is a proper authority to assume the obligation of the licensing process.

Registration: is the listing of an individual's name and other information on the official roster of a governmental agency. Nurses who are registered are permitted to use the title "Registered Nurses"

Certification: is the voluntary practice of validating that individual nurses met minimum standards of nursing competence in specialty areas such as pediatrics, mental health, gerontology and school health nursing.

Accreditation: is a process by which a voluntary organization or governmental agency appraises and grants accredited status to institutions and/or programs. The purpose of accreditation of programs in nursing is:

- To foster the continuous development and improvement in the quality of education in nursing
- To evaluate nursing programs in relation to the stated physiology and outcomes and to the established criteria for accreditation.

- To bring together practitioners, administrators, faculty, and students in an activity directed towards improving educational preparation for nursing practice.
- To provide an external peer review process.

KEYWORD

Self-regulation is the ability to control one's behavior, emotions, and thoughts in the pursuit of long-term goals.

Nursing Code of Ethics

A code of ethics is a formal declaration of a group's ideals and values that serve as rules and guidelines for the group's professional acts and notify the public of its commitment.

Generally speaking, codes of ethics are greater than legal requirements, and they can never be lower than the legal norms of the profession.

Purposes of code of ethics

NThe nursing code of ethics has the following purposes:

- To inform the public about the minimum standards of the profession and to help them understand professional nursing conduct.
- To provide a sign of the profession's commitments to the public it serves.
- To outline the major ethical considerations of the profession.
- To provide general guidelines for professional behavior.
- To guide the profession in self-regulation.
- To remind nurses of the special responsibility they assume when caring for the sick.

ICN CODE OF ETHICS

The need for nursing is Universal. Respect for life, human dignity, and human rights are fundamental to the nursing profession. It is not limited by nationality, ethnicity, faith, color, age, sex, politics, or socioeconomic standing.

Nurses provide health care services to the person, the family, and the community, and they coordinate these services with those of other connected organizations.

Responsibility & Accountability

- The fundamental responsibility of the nurse is fourfold: to promote health, prevent illness, restore health and to alleviate suffering.
- Nurses act in a manner consistent with their professional responsibilities and standards of practice.
- Nurses advocate practice environments conducive to safe, competent and ethical care.
- Nurses work in accordance with dependent, interdependent and collaborative functions of nursing.
- Nurses carefully handle nursing practice on specific ethical issues and resolve the ethical problems systematically.
- Nurses are accountable for their professional judgment and action.

Nurses and people

The primary obligation of the nurse is to those who require nursing care.

In providing care, the nurse fosters an environment in which the individual's values, customs, and spiritual beliefs are honored.

The nurse maintains the confidentiality of personal information and shares it with discretion.

Nurses and Practice

The nurse is responsible for nursing practice and maintaining competence through ongoing education. The nurse maintains the greatest feasible nursing care standards within the constraints of a particular setting.

When accepting and allocating responsibilities, the nurse makes decisions based on the individual's level of competence.

When operating in a professional role, nurses must always uphold personal conduct standards that reflect well on the profession.

Nurse and Society

The nurse shares with other citizens the responsibility for initiating and supporting actions to meet the health and social needs of the public.

Nurse and Co-workers

The nurse sustains a cooperative relationship with coworkers in nursing and other fields. The nurse takes appropriate action to safeguard the individual when his care is endangered by a co-worker or any other health personnel.

Nurse and the Profession

In determining and implementing desirable standards for nursing practice and nursing education, the nurse is primarily responsible.

The nurse is actively expanding her professional knowledge base.

Through the professional organization, the nurse contributes to the establishment and maintenance of equitable social and economic working conditions in nursing.

KEYWORD

Professional organization is a group that usually seeks to further a particular profession, the interests of individuals and organisations engaged in that profession, and the public interest.

Nursing code of ethics in Ethiopia

The Ethiopian nurses association (ENA) code of ethics for registered nurses comprises key elements of the code. It includes values, responsibility statements, and levels of guidance or actions.

1. Accountability and Responsibility

- The fundamental responsibility of the nurse is fourfold: to promote health, prevent illness, restore health and to alleviate suffering.
- Nurses act in a manner consistent with their professional responsibilities and standards of practice.
- Nurses advocate a practice environment that is conducive to safe, competent and ethical care.
- Nurses work in accordance with dependent, interdependent and collaborative functions of nursing.
- Nurses carefully handle nursing practice on specific ethical issues and resolve the ethical problems systematically.
- Nurses are accountable for their professional judgment and action.

2. Respect rights and dignity

- The nurse provides care, unrestricted by consideration of nationality, race, creed, color, age, sex, politics, religion or social status.
- The nurse respects the value, customs and spiritual beliefs of an individual.
- The nurse identifies the health needs of the client, helps them to express their concern and obtains appropriate information and service.
- Nurses apply and promote principles of equity and fairness to assist clients in receiving biased treatment and share of health services and resources proportional to their needs.

KEYWORD

Diagnostic procedures may also be used to help plan treatment, find out how well treatment is working, and make a prognosis.

3. Confidentiality

- Nurses safeguard the trust of the clients that information and health records in the context of professional relationship are shared outside the health care team only with the clients' permission or as legally required.
- Nurses maintain privacy during therapeutic and diagnostic procedures.

4. Advocacy:

- Nurses sustain a cooperative relationship with other health workers in team work.
- Nurses value health and well-being and assist persons to achieve their optimum level of health in a situation of normal health, illness, injury or in the process of dying.
- Nurses promote safety prevent intentional or unintentional harm and take appropriate action to safeguard the individuals when their care is endangered by a coworker or any other person.
- The Nurse respects acceptance or refusal rights of the patient during therapeutic and diagnostic procedures or research and learning situations up on clients.

5. Professional development

- The nurse plays the major role in determining and implementing desirable Standards of nursing practice and nursing education.

- The nurse should develop professionally through formal and non-formal continuing education
- The nurse should participate in professional organizations and advocate equitable social and economic working conditions.

KEYWORD

Organisational framework provides a structure for integrated financial planning, project tracking, reporting and monitoring of performance indicators.

Responsibilities of nurses for specific ethical issues

Patient's Bill of Rights

On February 6, 1973, the House of Delegates passed a statement on a patient's bill of rights. The American Hospital Association publishes a patient's bill of rights with the goal that compliance with these rights would lead to more effective patient care and improved patient and hospital organization satisfaction. When care is provided inside an organizational framework, the typical doctor-patient interaction takes on a new dimension. Legal precedent has held that the institution is also liable for the patient. In acknowledgment of these factors, these rights are affirmed. The patient's rights are as follows:

- The patient has a right to considerate and respect full care.
- The patient has the right to receive from his physician complete, up-to-date information regarding his diagnosis, treatment, and prognosis in language the patient may be expected to comprehend. When it is not medically advisable to provide such information to the patient, it should be provided to the patient's representative. He has the right to know the identity of the doctor in charge of coordinating his care.
- The patient has the right to receive from his physician, before the start of any procedure and/or treatment, the information essential to give informed consent. Except in emergency situations, such information for informed consent should include, but is not limited to, the exact operation and/or treatment, the medically relevant risks involved, and the expected duration of incapacity. If there are medically relevant alternatives to care or treatment, or if the patient asks for information on medical alternatives, the patient has the right to be informed of these options. Additionally, the patient has the right to know who is accountable for the operations and/or treatment.
- The patient has the right to refuse treatment to the degree

permitted by law and to be informed of the medical ramifications of his refusal.

- The patient has the right to complete confidentiality on his own medical care program. Case separation, consultation, examination, and treatment are private and should be performed discretely. Those who are not directly involved in his care must obtain his consent to be present.
- The patent has the right to expect that all communications and records pertaining to his care should be treated as confidential.
- The patient has the right to expect that, within its ability, the hospital will respond to their request for services in a reasonable manner. The hospital must provide an evaluation, service, or referral based on the severity of the patient's condition. When medically permissible, a patient may be transferred to another facility only after receiving thorough information and explanation of the reasons for the transfer and alternatives to it. Prior to transferring a patient, the receiving institution must accept the patient for transfer.
- The patient has the right to seek information regarding the hospital's relationships with other health care and educational institutions in relation to his care.
- The patient has the right to know, by name, if any professional relationships exist between the personnel who are treating him.
- The patient has the right to be informed if the hospital intends or performs human experimentation that will influence his care or treatment. The patient has the right to decline participation in such studies.
- The patient is entitled to reasonable continuity of care. He is entitled to know in advance what appointment times and physicians are available, as well as their locations. The patient has the right to expect that the hospital will provide a method for his physician or the physician's delegate to tell him of his continuing health care needs after discharge.
- Regardless of the method of payment, the patient has the right to see and receive an explanation of his charge.
- The patient is entitled to know what hospital rules and regulations govern his behavior as a patient.

KEYWORD

Educational institution is a place where people of different ages gain an education, including preschools, childcare, primary-elementary schools, secondary-high schools, and universities.

Ethical Issues related to Patients' Rights

1. Right to Truth

The right of patients to know the truth about their condition, prognosis, and treatment is an issue between the physician and the patient. The current tendency among physicians is toward greater candor. In the past, the professional necessity to protect the patient from potential physical or emotional harm that could be caused by awareness of a critical or terminal condition frequently trumped the moral obligation to communicate the truth, because the patient has the right to know and adjust to it. Due to their extensive interactions with patients, nurses frequently find it difficult to accept a physician's decision to withhold the truth about a patient's health.

Due to the contradiction between physicians' choices and nurses' personal feelings, it may be prudent for the health care team to meet in order to settle the issue and develop a unified approach to the patient.

KEYWORD

Refusing therapy refers to a situation where a person declines or rejects a recommended medical or therapeutic intervention.

2. Right to Refuse Treatment

Patients may refuse therapy for reasons sometimes known only to themselves, despite the fact that failure to get treatment may result in death. The issue of refusal of treatment may require a court decision. Frequently, courts conclude that patent holders cannot be compelled to take treatment. In the case of a juvenile, however, courts are likely to decide that parents cannot refuse treatment for any reason. Typically, the child is made a temporary ward of the court and treatment can begin.

It may be difficult for a nurse to comprehend a patient's decision to die instead of accepting care. However, nurses must respect a patient's right to individual and personal views and ideas and must not allow their own emotions to interfere with patient treatment. If nurses are unable to reconcile their ethical principles with those of their patients, they should request removal from the case in the patient's best interest.

3. Informed Consent

Legally and ethically, the question of informed consent applies to numerous health care facilities. Patients have the right to accurate and sufficient information regarding both major and small procedures, so that their consent to undergo them is based on reasonable expectations.

edical practitioners are responsible for communicating information about major surgeries and complex medical treatments. Prior to initiating even the most basic nursing treatments, nurses should tell their patients in terms the patients may comprehend the operations. This involves responding to any inquiries patients might have. The failure to get informed, written permission before performing a procedure may subject nurses and other health care professionals to legal action or disciplinary action by state regulatory agencies.

Because nurses spend significant time with patients, they are more likely to be aware of their patients' inquiries and concerns. Often, these concerns should be brought to the attention of attending physicians, who may be unaware of the problems because they see the patient's lass regularly.

Did you get it?

Psychosurgery has always been a controversial medical field. The modern history of psychosurgery begins in the 1880s under the Swiss psychiatrist Gottlieb Burckhardt.

4. Human Experimentation

The scientific and medical communities are primarily concerned with research and human experimentation. If, however, nursing care is required for the experimental subjects, then nurses are involved. In these situations, nurses' obligations and ethical considerations involve ensuring that their patients' safety and informed permission for participation in research investigations are protected.

In these cases, the nurses' duty as patient advocates may place them in direct conflict with research staff and supporting agencies as well as human subjects research committees.

5. Behavior Control

The issue of informed consent is crucial in any type of behavioral control; the use of medications or psychosurgery further complicates an already difficult subject.

The authority of society to determine what constitutes good or acceptable behavior remains controversial. The issue concerns both private and public conduct. In addition, it concerns whether individuals have the right to determine for themselves what constitutes appropriate personal conduct, or whether others may decide for them based on some other definition of appropriate personal conduct.

In this context, one of the ethical issues with which nurses may be faced is the issue of informed permission for therapies designed to manage behavior. Nurses may question whether patients who are candidates for medication therapy or psychotherapy are able and competent to provide informed consent, and whether they have the right to decline treatment.

Health-related Legal issues in Ethiopia

Along with the patients' bill of rights, below are certain health-related issues commonly seen in Ethiopia.

KEYWORD

Criminal abortion is the unlawful expulsion of the fetus by artificial means. It is a felony when any person advises, assists in or performs an abortion.

1. Abortion:

- The nurse shall assist the physician if she/he is sure that an abortion is performed for the purpose of saving the endangered life or health of women.
- The nurse shall not attempt or carry out an abortion.
- It is mandatory for the nurse to treat a patient who is suffering from the effect of a criminal abortion induced by another provided there is no physician in the health institution.
- The nurse shall report to the concerned authorities of criminal abortion in the absence of a physician.
- The nurse has all the right not to participate in all procedures of criminal abortion.

2. Euthanasia

- The nurse shall never assist; collaborate in taking life as an act of mercy even at the direct request of the patient or patient's relatives.

3. Death

- The nurse shall note the exact cessation of vital signs and notify the attending physician to pronounce death.
- The nurse shall give due respect to the deceased taking in to consideration religion and cultural aspects.
- A nurse shall participate in or assist a medical team in taking out organ from a cadaver provided there is written consent of a patient or relatives.

4. Suicide

- A nurse who is taking care of a patient with a suicidal tendency shall remove all items that facilitate suicide such as sharp instruments, ropes, belts, drugs and make sure that the outlets are graded.
- The nurse should not leave a suicidal patient alone.

KEYWORD

Fertilisation is the fusion of gametes to give rise to a new individual organism or offspring and initiate its development.

5. Organ Transplantation:

- The nurse shall involve in any organ transplantation procedure provided that the donor and recipient have a clear written agreement, the donor gives informed consent and he/she is not mentally ill at the time of consent.
- The nurse shall advocate the declaration of human rights in the organ transplantation procedure.
- The nurse shall have moral and professional rights to make ethical decisions to resolve the dilemma that arises from the procedure.

6. Fertility Matter:

- The nurse shall respect the autonomy of the client for contraception and other fertility matter including artificial fertilization
- The nurse shall have moral and professional rights to make ethical decisions in a situation of a dilemma for the same.
- The nurse shall have a responsibility to give information about the case

Areas of Potential Liabilities in Nursing

Crimes and torts

A crime is an act committed in violation of public (criminal) law and punishable by a fine and/ or imprisonment.

A crime does not have to be intended in order to be a crime. For example, a nurse may accidentally give a client an additional and lethal dose of narcotics to relieve discomfort.

Crimes could be felonies and / or misdemeanors.

- Felonies: a crime of a serious nature such as murder, armed robbery, second-degree murder. A crime is punished through criminal action by the state.
- A misdemeanor: is an offense of a less serious nature and is usually punished with a fine or short-term jail sentence or both. For example, a nurse who slaps a client's face could be charged with a misdemeanor

A Tort

Is a civil wrong committed against a person or a person's property? Torts are usually litigated in court by civil action between individuals.

Tort may be classified as intentional or unintentional:

Intentional tort includes fraud, invasion of privacy, libel and slander assault and battery and false imprisonment.

Fraud: false presentation of some fact with the intention that it will be acted up on by another person. Example, it is fraud for a nurse applying to a hospital for employment to fail to list two past employers for deceptive reasons when asked for five previous employers.

False imprisonment: is "unlawful restraint or detention of another person against his or her wishes"

KEYWORD

Employment is a relationship between two parties regulating the provision of paid labour services.

Potential Malpractice Situation in Nursing

To avoid charges of malpractice, nurses need to recognize those nursing situation in which negligent actions are most likely to occur and to take measures to prevent them

The most common malpractice situations are

1. Medication error:

Which resulted from:

- Failing to read the medication label.
- Misunderstanding or incorrectly calculating the dose.
- Failing to identify the client correctly.
- Preparing the wrong concentration or
- Administration by the wrong route (e.g. Intravenously instead of intramuscularly)

TIPS

Dicumarol is a naturally occurring anticoagulant drug that depletes stores of vitamin K. It is also used in biochemical experiments as an inhibitor of reductases.

Some errors are serious and can result in death. For example, administration of Decumarol to a client who recently returned from surgery could cause the client to have a hemorrhage.

2. Sponges or other small items can be left inside a client during an operation.
3. Burning a client: May be caused by hot water bottles, heating pads, and solutions that are too hot for applications.
4. Clients often fall accidentally: As a result that a nurse leaves the rails down or leaves a baby unattended on a bath table.
5. Ignoring a client's complaints .
6. Incorrectly identifying clients
7. Loss of client's property: jewelry, money, eye glasses and dentures.

MEASURES TO PREVENT THE ABOVE MALPRACTICE SITUATIONS.

- A nurse always needs to check and recheck medications very carefully before administering a drug.
- The surgical team should count correctly before the surgeon closes the incision.

Reporting Crimes, Torts and Unsafe Practice

A nurse may need to report nursing colleagues or other health professionals for practices that endanger the health and safety of a client. For example, Alcohol and drug use theft from a client or agency, and unsafe nursing practice.

Guidelines for reporting a crime, tort or unsafe practices are:

- Write a clear description of a situation you believe you should report.
- Make sure that your statements are accurate
- Make sure you are credible
- Obtain support from at least one trust worth person before filing the report.
- Report the matter starting at the lowest possible level in the agency hierarchy.

- Assume responsibility for reporting the individual by being open about it, sign your name to the letter.
- See the problem through once you have reported it.

KEYWORD

Team communication extends beyond that basic two-person interaction to encompass the exchange of information between any number of individuals in your business.

Record Keeping

Reporting and Documenting

Reporting: oral or written account of patient status; between members of the health care team. Reports should be clear, concise, and comprehensive.

Documenting: patient record/chart provides written documentation of the patient's status and treatment

Purpose: continuity of care, legal document, research, statistics, education, audits

What to document: assessment, plan of care, nursing interventions (care, teaching, safety measures), outcome of care, change in status, health care team communication,

Characteristics of documentation: brief, concise, comprehensive, factual, descriptive, objective, relevant/appropriate, legally prudent

Record Keeping

- Health records are the means by which information is communicated about clients and means of ensuring continuity of care.
- The clients' medical record is a legal document and can be produced in a court as evidence.
- Records are used as risk management tools and for research purposes.
- Often the record is used to remind a witness of events surrounding a lawsuit, because several months or years usually elapse before the suit goes to trial.
- The effectiveness of the record depends upon the accuracy and completeness of the record.
- Nurses need to keep accurate and complete records of nursing care provided to clients.

Insufficient or inaccurate documentation:

- Can constitute negligence and be the basis for tort liability.
- Hinder proper diagnosis and treatment and result in injury to the client.

Accurate Record keeping

- Routine nursing assessment and intervention should be documented properly.
- Use a pen rather than a pencil during documentation.
- When making a correction do not raise the previous draw one line on an old and add correction so the previous remained legible because correction is not for changing.
- Write legibly.
- Document all information.
- Add time, date, name and other important information.
- Document all medically related conditions.
- Use specific terms.
- Statements should not be biased.

The Incident Report

KEYWORD

Statistical data are the outcomes or the observations which occur in scientific experiments or an investigation.

An incident report is an agency record of an accident or incident.

Whenever a patient is injured or has a potential injury there exists a possibility of a lawsuit, such a report must be recorded.

An incidental report may be written for situations involving a patient, visitors, or employee.

The incident report used to:

- To make all the facts about an accident available to personnel
- To contribute to statistical data about accidents or incidents.
- To help health personnel to prevent future accidents.

Information to include in the incident report

- Identify the client by name and hospitals
- Give the date and time of the incident. Avoid any conclusions

or blame. Describe the incident as you saw it even if your impressions differ from those of others

- Identify all witnesses to the incident
- Identify any equipment by number and any medication by name and number.
- Document any circumstance surrounding the incident. For example, that another client is experiencing cardiac arrest.

Remember

The reports should be completed as soon as possible i.e., within 24 hours of the incident and filed according to agencies policy.

Wills

A will is a declaration by a person about how the person's property or cash is to be disposed/ distributed after death.

In order for a will to be valid the following conditions must be met:

- The person making the will should be mentally conscious
- The person should not be unduly influenced by anyone else.

A nurse may be required to witness a will. A will must be signed in the presence of two witnesses.

When witnessing a will, the nurse

- Attests that the client signed a document that is stated to be the client's last will.
- Attests that the client appears to be mentally sound and appreciates the significance of their action.

If a nurse witnesses a will, the nurse should record on the client's card that the will was made and the patient's physical and mental condition.

Remember

If a nurse does not wish to act as a witness. For example, if a nurse's opinion undue influence has been brought on the client- then it is the nurse's right to refuse to act in this capacity.

Use of Recording

- Provides accurate information for later use.
- May be useful if the will is contested

Euthanasia

It is the act of pennilessly putting to death persons suffering from incurable or distressing diseases. It is commonly referred as "mercy killing"

Types of Euthanasia

- ***Active euthanasia***: is a deliberate attempt to end life. e.g., deprivation of oxygen supply, administering an agent that would result in death.
- ***Passive euthanasia***: allowing death by withdrawing or withholding treatment. No special attempt will be made to revive the patient

All forms of euthanasia are illegal except in states where the right to die status and living will exist.

REVIEW QUESTIONS

1. Define ethics and identify its relation and difference with that of morality.
2. What are the common principles of ethics and their similarity and deference?
3. What are the nursing practice act, the standard of practice, and code of ethics?
4. When and how do nurses hold in confidence and in private any information obtained during their professional performance?
5. What is the basic characteristics and advantage of documentation?

MULTIPLE CHOICE QUESTIONS

1. Which statement would best explain the role of the nurse when planning care for a culturally diverse population? The nurse will plan care to:

a. Include care that is culturally congruent with the staff from predetermined criteria
b. Focus only on the needs of the client, ignoring the nurse's beliefs and practices
c. Blend the values of the nurse that are for the good of the client and minimize the client's individual values and beliefs during care
d. Provide care while aware of one's own bias, focusing on the client's individual needs rather than the staff's practices

2. Which factor is *least* significant during assessment when gathering information about cultural practices?

a. Language, timing
b. Touch, eye contact
c. Biocultural needs
d. Pain perception, management expectations

3. Transcultural nursing implies:

a. Using a comparative study of cultures to understand similarities and differences across human groups to provide specific individualized care that is culturally appropriate
b. Working in another culture to practice nursing within their limitations
c. Combining all cultural beliefs into a practice that is a non-threatening approach to minimize cultural barriers for all clients' equality of care
d. Ignoring all cultural differences to provide the best generalized care to all clients.

4. What should the nurse do when planning nursing care for a client with a different cultural background? The nurse should:

a. Allow the family to provide care during the hospital stay so no rituals or customs are broken
b. Identify how these cultural variables affect the health problem

c. Speak slowly and show pictures to make sure the client always understands

d. Explain how the client must adapt to hospital routines to be effectively cared for while in the hospital

5. Which activity would not be expected by the nurse to meet the cultural needs of the client?

a. Promote and support attitudes, behaviors, knowledge, and skills to respectfully meet client's cultural needs despite the nurse's own beliefs and practices

b. Ensure that the interpreter understands not only the language of the client but feelings and attitudes behind cultural practices to make sure an ethical balance can be achieved

c. Develop structure and process for meeting cultural needs on a regular basis and means to avoid overlooking these needs with clients

d. Expect the family to keep an interpreter present at all times to assist in meeting the communication needs all day and night while hospitalized

Answers to Multiple Choice Questions

1. (d) 2. (c) 3. (a) 4.(b) 5.(d)

REFERENCES

1. Burkhardt A, and Nathaniel A., Ethical issues in contemporary nursing. 2nd edition, 2002, Delmar publishers, USA.
2. Canadian nursing Association, Every day ethics: Putting the code in to practice, 1997, Ottawa, Canada.
3. Ethiopian Nurses association, Standard of Nursing in Ethiopia, 2002 (Draft Document).
4. Ethiopian Nurses association, Code of Ethics Nursing in Ethiopia, 2002 (Draft Document).
5. Gloria M., Nursing perspectives and issues, 3rd edition, 1986 Delmar publishers Inc.
6. Jorge Grimes and Elizabeth, Health assessment in nursing practice, 4th edition, 1996, Little, Brown and Company, Boston.
7. Hein C. Communication in nursing practice, 1990, Little, Brown and company
8. Kozier, B. ERB, G., Blais, K., Wilkinson. J., Leuven, K., Fundamentals of Nursing: Concepts, processes and practices, 5th edition, 1998, Addison Weskley Longman, Inc, California.
9. Kay Kittrell Chitty, Professional Nursing: Concepts and challenges, 2nd edition, 1993, W.B. Sounders company Philadelphia. Ministry of Health, Ethiopia,
10. Purtilo and Cassel., Ethical Dimensions in the health professions, 1st edition W.B. Sounders company, Philadelphia,

11. Tayler C. Carol Lillis and Priscilla L., Fundamentals of nursing the art and science of nursing, 1999, care.J.b. Lippincott Company.
12. Airth-Kindree, N, M, M., &Kirkhorn, L, C. (2016). Ethical Grand Rounds: Teaching Ethics at the Point of Care. *Nursing Education Perspectices, 37*(1), 48-50. doi: 10.5480/13-1128
13. Bratz,J, K, A., & Sandoval-Ramirez, M. (2017). Ethical competences for the development og nursing care. *Thematic issue: Education and teaching in Nursing.* DOI: http://dx.doi.org/10.1590/0034-7167-2017-0539
14. Chadwick, R., Tadd, W., & Gallagher, A. (2016). *Ethics and Nursing Profession.* London: Palgrave. Retrieved from https://books.google.com.au/books?hl=en&lr=&id=vG6CDAAAQBAJ&oi=fnd&pg=PP1&dq=autonomy+ethical+principles+in+nursing&ots=_JgdqZD0fi&sig=bijGcOa0aCwRfnlioVeba6Om22Q&redir_esc=y#v=onepage&q=autonomy%20ethical%20principles%20in%20nursing&f=false
15. Doody, O., &Noonam, M. (2016). Nursing research ethics, guidance and application in practice. *British Journal of Nursing. 25*(14). Doi: https://doi.org/10.12968/bjon.2016.25.14.803
16. Ellis, P. (2017). *Understanding Ethics for Nursing Students.* Sage Publication. Retrieved from https://books.google.com.au/books?hl=en&lr=&id=SiElDwAAQBAJ&oi=fnd&pg=PP1&dq=autonomy+ethical+principles+in+nursing&ots=tGlpPDzFXr&sig=_8a7_NAUU8nvdV1lY394ljCvmU0&redir_esc=y#v=onepage&q=autonomy%20ethical%20principles%20in%20nursing&f=false
17. Epstein, B., & Turner, M. (2015). The Nursing Code of Ethics: Its Value, Its History. *Online Journal of Issues in Nursing. 20*(2), 4. doi: 10.3912/OJIN.Vol20No02Man04
18. Haddad, L, M., & Geiger, R, A. (2019). Nursing Ethical Considerations. *Treaseure Island (FL): StatPearls Publishing.* Retrieved from https://www.ncbi.nlm.nih.gov/books/NBK526054/
19. Hain, J, D., Diaz, D., &Paixao, R. (2016). What are Ethical Issues When Honoring an Older Adult's Decision to Withdraw from Dialysis?. *Nephrology Nursing Journal. 43*(5), 429-450. Retrieved from https://web.a.ebscohost.com/ehost/pdfviewer/pdfviewer?vid=1&sid=b62f8380-9f8f-4cc5-9023-2ec5e85ef1cd%40sessionmgr4006
20. Kangasniemi, M., Korhonen, A., &Pakkanen, P. (2015). Professional ethics in nursing: An integrative review. *Journal of Advanced Nursing, 71*(8) doi:10.1111/jan.12619
21. National Commission on Correctional Health Care. (2019). *Ethical and Legal Issues.* Retrieved from https://www.ncchc.org/cnp-ethical-legal
22. Nursing and Midwifery Board of Australia, (2016). *Code of Ethics for Nurses in Australia.* Retrieved from https://www.nursingmidwiferyboard.gov.au/Codes-Guidelines-Statements/Professional-standards.aspx
23. Nursing and Midwifery Board of Australia, (2016). *Code of conduct for nurses.* Retrieved from https://www.nursingmidwiferyboard.gov.au/Codes-Guidelines-Statements/Professional-standards.aspx

24. Nursing and Midewifery Board of Australia, (2016). *Registered Nurses Standards for Practice.* Retrieved from https://www.nursingmidwiferyboard.gov.au/Codes-Guidelines-Statements/Professional-standards.aspx
25. Schick-Makaroff, K., &Storch, J, L. (2019). Guidance for Ethical Leadership in Nursing Codes of Ethics: An Integrative Review. *Nursing Research. 32*(1), 60-73. Retrieved from https://web.a.ebscohost.com/ehost/pdfviewer/pdfviewer?vid=1&sid=5fbe029d-b506-41ba-af91-be3fdf16315b%40sessionmgr4008
26. Tsuruwaka, M. (2017). Consulted ethical problems of clinical nursing practice: perspectice of faculty members in Japan. *BMC Nursing. 16*(23). Doi: 10.1186/s12912-017-0217-3

INDEX

C